COPING WITH POLYCYSTIC OVARY SYNDROME

CHRISTINE CRAGGS-HINTON, mother of three, followed a career in the Civil Service until, in 1991, she
developed fibromyalgia, a chronic pain condition. Christine took up writing for therapeutic reasons, and has, in the
last few years, produced *Living with Fibromyalgia*, *The
Fibromyalgia Healing Diet* and *The Chronic Fatigue
Healing Diet* (all published by Sheldon Press). She also
writes for the Fibromyalgia Association UK and the
related *FaMily* magazine. In recent years she has become
interested in fiction writing, too.

ADAM BALEN is Consultant in Reproductive Medicine
and Surgery at Leeds General Infirmary, where he
participates in the management of an IVF unit. The author
of five books, including *The Practical Management of
Polycystic Ovary Syndrome*, he has also written numerous
articles and chapters on a variety of areas related to
reproductive medicine for journals and edited collections.
He has had a particular interest in the causes and
management of polycystic ovary syndrome for many
years.

Overcoming Common Problems Series

Selected titles

A full list of titles is available from Sheldon Press,
1 Marylebone Road, London NW1 4DU, and on our website at
www.sheldonpress.co.uk

Assertiveness: Step by Step
Dr Windy Dryden and Daniel Constantinou

Body Language at Work
Mary Hartley

Cancer – A Family Affair
Neville Shone

The Cancer Guide for Men
Helen Beare and Neil Priddy

The Candida Diet Book
Karen Brody

The Chronic Fatigue Healing Diet
Christine Craggs-Hinton

Cider Vinegar
Margaret Hills

Comfort for Depression
Janet Horwood

Confidence Works
Gladeana McMahon

Considering Adoption?
Sarah Biggs

Coping Successfully with Hay Fever
Dr Robert Youngson

Coping Successfully with Pain
Neville Shone

Coping Successfully with Panic Attacks
Shirley Trickett

Coping Successfully with Prostate Cancer
Dr Tom Smith

Coping Successfully with Prostate Problems
Rosy Reynolds

Coping Successfully with RSI
Maggie Black and Penny Gray

Coping Successfully with Your Hiatus Hernia
Dr Tom Smith

Coping When Your Child Has Special Needs
Suzanne Askham

Coping with Alopecia
Dr Nigel Hunt and Dr Sue McHale

Coping with Anxiety and Depression
Shirley Trickett

Coping with Blushing
Dr Robert Edelmann

Coping with Bronchitis and Emphysema
Dr Tom Smith

Coping with Candida
Shirley Trickett

Coping with Childhood Asthma
Jill Eckersley

Coping with Chronic Fatigue
Trudie Chalder

Coping with Coeliac Disease
Karen Brody

Coping with Cystitis
Caroline Clayton

Coping with Depression and Elation
Dr Patrick McKeon

Coping with Eczema
Dr Robert Youngson

Coping with Endometriosis
Jo Mears

Coping with Epilepsy
Fiona Marshall and
Dr Pamela Crawford

Coping with Fibroids
Mary-Claire Mason

Coping with Gallstones
Dr Joan Gomez

Coping with a Hernia
Dr David Delvin

Coping with Incontinence
Dr Joan Gomez

Coping with Long-Term Illness
Barbara Baker

Coping with the Menopause
Janet Horwood

Coping with Polycystic Ovary Syndrome
Christine Craggs-Hinton

Coping with Psoriasis
Professor Ronald Marks

Coping with Rheumatism and Arthritis
Dr Robert Youngson

Coping with SAD
Fiona Marshall and Peter Cheevers

Overcoming Common Problems Series

Overcoming Common Problems Series

Overcoming Common Problems

Coping with Polycystic Ovary Syndrome

Christine Craggs-Hinton
and
Dr Adam Balen

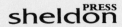

First published in Great Britain in 2004 by
Sheldon Press
1 Marylebone Road
London NW1 4DU

British Library Cataloguing-in-Publication Data

A catalogue record for this book is available from the British Library

ISBN 0–85969–908–0

1 3 5 7 9 10 8 6 4 2

Typeset by Deltatype Limited, Birkenhead, Merseyside
Printed in Great Britain by Biddles Ltd
www.biddles.co.uk

Contents

Authors' Note

This book was written by Christine Craggs-Hinton. Invaluable input into the scientific and medical chapters was given by Adam Balen, MB, BS, MD, FRCOG, consultant obstetrician and gynaecologist and specialist in reproductive medicine and surgery, and medical advisor for Verity, the support group for people with polycystic ovary syndrome. Adam Balen has also checked and approved the full content.

Foreword

Polycystic ovary syndrome (PCOS) is the commonest hormonal disturbance to affect women. As a syndrome the condition encompasses a wide range of features that can cause a variety of problems at different times in a woman's life. The symptoms may be severe for some women and relatively mild for others – to the extent that they have been put down by some doctors as being what can be expected as 'normal'. There has, therefore, been confusion among some doctors about making the diagnosis and about the best way to manage the various problems that are experienced.

It is important if you have PCOS that you have an understanding of the condition, what it may mean in the short term with respect to the problems that you may be experiencing and also in the long term regarding your general health. There are now a number of excellent support groups and useful websites that provide information. But do remember that not everything that you may read necessarily applies to you. As an individual you require a personal approach to your problems and so you may need to see a doctor who has a full understanding of your situation. There are also many steps that you can take in order to improve things for yourself.

Lifestyle matters! There is no doubt that an increase in body weight leads to a worsening of many of the symptoms of PCOS. As a society we now eat more than we were designed to and exercise less. Some women are predestined by their genes to have PCOS. Our genes determine how our body works and how it behaves in different circumstances. There are probably many genes that are involved in the development of PCOS: some may result in changes in body weight, others in hormone production by the ovaries and others in the way the body responds to different hormones. The expression of the syndrome will depend on the particular combination of genes that are active and also on other factors, such as diet, activity and racial differences.

In *Coping with PCOS* we provide an overview of the syndrome that aims to cover all aspects of the condition in an easy-to-understand manner. We deal with the various aspects of PCOS and

ix

how they are investigated and treated, both medically and by lifestyle and dietary adaptations.

We hope that you find the book informative and helpful. If you feel that there are issues that we have not covered then we shall be happy to hear from you. Although we shall not be able to answer specific questions directly, we shall try to address them in future editions.

Adam Balen

Introduction

Polycystic ovary syndrome (PCOS) is a common condition, yet many doctors are not sufficiently enlightened about it to be able to make a diagnosis readily. It seems that this unfortunate fact is then compounded by women failing to describe all their symptoms at the consultation. It is easy to understand why, too, given that they are likely to experience such seemingly unrelated problems as facial hair, acne and irregular periods. Not the easiest things to talk about either.

The symptoms of this complex condition are caused by a hormonal imbalance. There are a variety of approaches to treatment, which may differ over time depending on the needs of the individual patient. Practitioners of orthodox medicine frequently advise taking the contraceptive pill and perhaps other hormone preparations, which can work to great effect and are discussed in this book. However, these therapies do not provide a cure. Fortunately, great improvements may also be made by more natural means, and this book attempts to discuss them all, from diet and lifestyle changes to advice on how to improve your self-image, how to get the most from your relationships and how to reduce stress.

1

What Is Polycystic Ovary Syndrome?

Polycystic ovary syndrome, known as PCOS, is the most common endocrine (hormonal) disorder in women of reproductive age. It is characterized by a collection of symptoms, which include:

- excessive facial and/or body hair (hirsutism),
- weight gain,
- adult acne or excessively oily skin,
- absent or irregular periods,
- difficulty getting pregnant,
- hair loss (alopecia).

The other symptoms that may be associated with PCOS include:

- mood swings,
- tender breasts,
- miscarriage,
- bloating,
- fatigue,
- joint pain,
- depression,
- pelvic or abdominal pain.

In addition, women with PCOS are at greater risk of developing some longer-term health problems. They include:

- late-onset (type 2) diabetes,
- high cholesterol levels, heart disease and stroke,
- cancer of the lining of the womb (endometrium).

The main problems experienced by women with PCOS are menstrual cycle disturbances (irregular or absent periods), difficulty controlling body weight, and skin problems (acne and unwanted hair growth on the face or body). Not all women with PCOS experience all of the symptoms and a woman's problems may change over time. In particular, if a person with PCOS becomes overweight then her problems will worsen.

About 30 per cent of all women have multiple cysts on their ovaries, although a smaller proportion will have symptoms of PCOS. 'Polycystic' means 'many cysts', and 'syndrome' indicates a collection of more than one symptom. Not all of the above symptoms need necessarily occur together in PCOS.

The condition was first described by Irving Stein and Michael Leventhal in 1935.[1] In fact, until fairly recently it was known as Stein–Leventhal syndrome. Because it was not possible in the 1930s to carry out the hormone blood tests and ultrasound scans that we take for granted today, the diagnosis was then based on absent periods, hirsutism and obesity. The combination of these three symptoms are now seen as the classic features of PCOS. However, it is clear that the syndrome comes with a wide spectrum of possible symptoms, which, unfortunately, can make diagnosis difficult.

Table 1: Frequency of symptoms in women with PCOS

Symptom	Percentage
Irregular periods (oligomenorrhoea)	60–90
Excessive facial or body hair (hirsutism)	70–80
Infertility	40–60
Being overweight (obesity)	30–50
Absence of periods (amenorrhoea)	30–50
Acne	20–35

Various studies have shown certain symptom patterns in women with PCOS (Table 1). As you can see from the table, irregular periods appear to be the most common symptom, closely followed by hirsutism, infertility and being overweight.

If one looks at statistics in another way, it is clear that, among women with irregular periods about 80–90 per cent have PCOS, among women with acne about 90 per cent have PCOS, and among women with hirsutism about 95 per cent have PCOS.

Irregular or absent periods

A 'regular' menstrual cycle is defined as being between 23 and 35 days from the start of one period to the start of the next; in addition, a 'regular' cycle does not vary by more than 2 days on either side of its average length. If your own menstrual cycle, from the day you start one period to the day you start your next period, varies by more than that it can be classed as irregular; similarly, it is irregular if the frequency of your periods is less than 23 or more than 35 days.

A cycle of longer than 35 days is known as oligomenorrhoea (infrequent menses), whereas 6 months or more without a period is known as amenorrhoea (absent menses). In women who have oligomenorrhoea, ovulation – the release of the egg from the ovary – may either be irregular or not take place at all. As you read on, you will see that this situation can be controlled by the use of the contraceptive pill, which is of most benefit to women who also require a good form of contraception. Preparations of the hormone progesterone may also be used to help to regulate the cycle. (See Chapter 3 for details of medications that help to regulate menstruation.) Irregular or absent periods may also, in some cases, be controlled by more natural means, which are outlined in Chapters 5 and 6.

Hirsutism

Hirsutism, an embarrassing condition, is defined as excessive facial or body hair, or both. The distribution is commonly in a male pattern, the possible areas affected being the upper lip, chin, upper and lower back, chest, upper and lower abdomen, upper arm, thighs and buttocks.

The problem can be treated by the use of chemical depilatory creams, bleaching, laser, electrolysis, waxing and shaving. If you do not want to become pregnant, your doctor may prescribe the contraceptive pill – often Dianette or Yasmin – to reduce the growth of unwanted hair. As this type of therapy can take many months to show benefits, the hair removal techniques mentioned above may be used in the mean time. (See Chapter 3 for more details of the medications that treat hirsutism, and Chapter 5 for further information on hair removal techniques.)

Infertility

Fertility depends on many factors. For a start, ovulation – the release of the egg from the ovary – must occur, the male partner's sperm need to function normally, and the sperm require a normal passage to reach the Fallopian tubes, where fertilization takes place. It is a fact, though, that fertility declines with increasing age – particularly the age of the female partner. Investigations are usually started after a couple have been trying to get pregnant for a year, since by this time it is expected that about 85 per cent of young couples (under the age of 30) should have conceived. If there is an obvious reason for reduced fertility (for example, infrequent menstrual periods and therefore few ovulations), it is reasonable to start investigations and treatment straight away.

The irregular ovulation often seen in PCOS is the most common reason for pregnancy being difficult to achieve. A woman normally releases an egg once a month and can conceive at this time. When the number of times she ovulates is reduced, the number of times she can become pregnant is also reduced. However, there are several medications that can effectively kick-start the ovaries into action, and they are discussed in Chapters 3 and 4.

Sadly, women with PCOS do appear to have a tendency to miscarry. Recurrent miscarriage (that is three or more miscarriages) has also been linked with PCOS. The exact cause is often unknown but may be related to hormonal disturbances and being overweight. Weight loss in overweight women with PCOS can dramatically improve their chances of getting pregnant and continuing the pregnancy to term.

Normal function of the ovaries and what happens in PCOS are described in detail in Chapter 2.

Being overweight

Weight management problems are common in PCOS, with some sufferers putting on extra kilograms from puberty, when the female sex hormones can first go awry. A normal body mass index is between 20 and 25 kg/m^2 (calculated by taking the weight in kilograms and dividing it by the square of height in metres), but women with PCOS are often heavier than that. Unfortunately, weight gain can be a double-edged sword in PCOS. Women with polycystic ovaries who would not normally develop the syndrome

4

can start having symptoms when they become overweight. And since a woman with PCOS may have a slower metabolism than normal, weight loss can be hard to achieve.

Although there is no particular pattern of fat distribution for some women with PCOS, many others put on weight around their middle. Consequently, the ratio of the measurement around the waist to the measurement around the hips is often increased. This is commonly known as being 'apple-shaped' as opposed to 'pear-shaped'.

Unfortunately, being overweight worsens the symptoms of PCOS – especially acne, unwanted hair and infertility. Weight reduction will generally improve control of the menstrual cycle, reduce the heaviness of the menstrual flow and improve fertility and the other symptoms of PCOS. A healthy eating plan combined with aerobic exercise is the only real answer (for more information about diet and exercise, see Chapter 5). However, some drug therapies may also help (see Chapter 3). Try to enlist the support of not only your doctor, but also of your family and friends. Ask to be referred to a dietician if you feel you are unable to follow the diet recommended in this book.

Acne

Acne (spots on the face and body) is common in teenagers. However, when this problem persists into adult life (beyond the age of 20) the most common cause is PCOS. Acne and an excessively oily skin are largely a result of the raised testosterone levels in PCOS. Testosterone has an effect on the sebaceous glands, which lubricate the skin, and causes them to go into overdrive, producing relatively large amounts of oil, which clogs up the pores (the tiny tunnels leading to the skin surface). Everyone has bacteria that normally exist on the surface of the skin, but when the pores become blocked the bacteria multiply within the sebaceous gland and spots and small cysts appear. Acne can appear on the chest and back as well as on the face.

Over-the-counter creams and lotions may be of some use in treating acne, as may the long-term use of antibiotics (erythromycin and tetracyclines – although tetracyclines must not be taken if you are trying to get pregnant). However, these products will not treat the underlying hormone imbalance that causes the acne in the first place. Again, if you do not wish to get pregnant, your doctor may prescribe a contraceptive pill, such as Dianette or Yasmin, which has the additional benefit of acne reduction.

Unfortunately, some women have reported a worsening of their acne when they discontinue taking the contraceptive pill. Whether you use this type of medication or not, the best long-term option is probably an improved diet (see Chapter 5) and drinking lots of water. Some people find regular use of tea tree oil or hemp oil effective. These oils are applied directly to the skin. (For more information on the medications that are used to treat acne, see Chapter 3.)

An embarrassing condition

Women with PCOS can find themselves having to deal with a whole host of embarrassing symptoms. It is one thing to visit your doctor because you feel under the weather, quite another to visit your doctor because you have hairy nipples and facial hair. Most women believe that a tendency to excess facial or body hair is something they were born with. They are surprised to learn that it can be a symptom of hormonal disturbances and that, therefore, it is treatable. It is the same with persistent adult acne. Women tend to think it is 'just one of those things', that they have drawn the short straw where spots are concerned and that it is just a matter of trying to come to terms with them.

Furthermore, who wants to see the doctor because they've been putting on weight? Surely, if they're not laughed out of the surgery they'll be told to stop eating so much. Being overweight can be embarrassing, not least because onlookers jump to the conclusion that you have been overeating – in other words, indulging yourself. Conversely, sudden weight loss is another matter entirely. Not only are family and friends terribly concerned, doctors are too.

Frequently, when women tell their doctors that their periods are irregular, this problem is treated in isolation. The reason is generally because women don't even think to mention unwanted hair, acne and an increase in weight – what can these other problems possibly have to do with irregular periods? It is a fact, though, that the doctor needs to see the whole picture before he or she can make a correct diagnosis. The doctor cannot know, just by looking at you, that you use a depilatory cream every week and wouldn't be seen dead without doing so.

In the same way, your doctor will have no way of knowing that you've tried every diet you've ever been able to lay your hands on, but to no avail. It is also possible, if the doctor gives you only a cursory glance, that he or she won't realize that you have acne beneath all that concealing foundation. Forgive us if you personally don't suffer from these particular symptoms, but you will see what we mean. PCOS is not the easiest condition for either the patient or the doctor to recognize.

In many cases, the doctor may consider symptoms of hair loss, weight gain, fatigue, irritability and irregular periods as indicators of stress, for stress is known to have wide-ranging effects. Alternatively, mood swings, fatigue, pelvic and abdominal pain and irregular periods may be attributed to premenstrual syndrome (PMS). With a condition that is as difficult to diagnose as PCOS, the patient herself may have to do some of the groundwork and then bring the condition to her doctor's attention. Unfortunately, in the end the responsibility of our own health lies with us and not with our doctors.

A condition to be taken seriously

To continue on the subject of embarrassing symptoms, some women are even reluctant to inform the doctor that their periods are irregular. Many of us were brought up believing that periods are 'the curse' and that they naturally cause moodiness, pelvic and abdominal pain and even acne. Those with scanty periods may see the doctor, only to be told they should think themselves lucky, that a light flow is far easier to deal with than a heavier one. But unfortunately, long gaps between periods can lead to abnormal thickening of the womb lining, and this in turn can increase the risk of endometrial cancer. It is essential therefore to ensure that the lining of the womb is shed at least once every 3 months to prevent abnormal thickening. Scanty or irregular periods are not always a symptom of PCOS, but they usually are.

The trouble with PCOS is that, if it is left untreated, the long-term health risks mentioned earlier may eventually rear their ugly heads. These health risks are discussed in more detail in Chapter 2.

Unfortunately, infertility is also a serious shorter-term knock-on effect experienced by some sufferers. Women tend to expect to have little or no trouble getting pregnant and so generally put off trying to conceive until the time is right – after all, pregnancy and ultimately childbirth are perhaps the most natural female functions of all. However, when there is no sign of a pregnancy after months or even years of trying ... well, it can feel like the end of the world. Infertility problems can cause great heartache. There are solutions, however – as you will find as you read on.

What does it feel like to suffer from PCOS?

Although the symptoms of PCOS vary a great deal from person to person, sufferers often complain of feeling tired. They are likely to be concerned about their periods – as noted above, the periods are either heavy and frequent, scant and infrequent, or non-existent. Consequently, they may worry about their ability to have children. Excessive facial or body hair, acne and weight gain often arise in puberty, but women can develop symptoms in their 20s, 30s and even into their 40s. Also, because many of the symptoms rate high on the embarrassment scale, the woman will doubtlessly find her confidence shaken. It can be frightening, too, to develop such symptoms seemingly out of the blue.

When hair loss from the head is a problem as well as hair growth in a male pattern on the face and body, some women are even secretly afraid they are turning into men. To feel your femininity threatened in such a way can be nothing less than terrifying. It doesn't even take hair loss for some women to feel they are losing their femininity – putting on weight, developing acne and growing unwanted hair can have the same effect. Obviously, this can lead to psychological problems.

The fact that some doctors may at first find nothing wrong, or attribute the symptoms to stress doesn't help matters, either. Then, when a correct diagnosis is finally achieved, there can be mixed feelings of relief and fear at what may lie ahead. However, please feel assured that medications, lifestyle adjustments and stress management techniques can make an enormous difference in PCOS.

The emotional aspects of PCOS are discussed in Chapter 7.

Can the cysts in PCOS be removed?

It is a misconception that the ovarian cysts themselves are the cause of PCOS. They are, in fact, a result of the hormonal disturbances within the ovary. In PCOS the ovarian follicles do not develop normally, and ovulation fails to occur on a regular basis, which is why the little follicles or cysts remain in the ovary and can be clearly seen on an ultrasound scan. In PCOS the cysts themselves are very small – measuring only 2–8 mm ($\frac{1}{12}$–$\frac{1}{3}$ inch) in diameter, and there are usually ten or so around the ovary perimeter. Removal of the cysts is not helpful, however, for that would fail to resolve the hormonal imbalance. In fact, if they were cut away, more cysts would form.

What are generally referred to as 'ovarian cysts' are different from the cysts in PCOS in that they are usually single and can grow to a much greater size (perhaps 30 mm ($1\frac{1}{5}$ inches) or more). A woman with PCOS has as much chance as one with normal ovaries of developing a very large ovarian cyst. If this occurs, it may require surgical removal.

Is PCOS curable?

Although PCOS is a malfunction of the body that cannot be permanently 'cured', it should not be regarded as a disease. The symptoms can be controlled with medical treatments combined with the right lifestyle changes and, perhaps, complementary therapies. As a result, your life can become far more productive, in every sense of the word. Instead of telling yourself you have an incurable condition, try to think of it as an ongoing health concern requiring long-term treatment.

2

What Causes Polycystic Ovary Syndrome?

PCOS is a complex disorder in which the function of the ovaries is affected and the body's metabolism may be disturbed. A condition known as 'insulin resistance' is also likely to be present.

It appears there are many factors that can predispose a woman to the development of PCOS, including familial (that is genetic) links, environmental factors (for example, diet affecting body weight) and imbalances in the production of hormones from the various glands (the ovaries, the adrenal glands, the pancreas and the pituitary). Lifestyle and environmental factors can also play a role in either triggering or worsening the condition (see Chapter 5).

The cause and course of the condition has been examined in some well-documented studies.[2, 3]

A familial link

By investigating large families, researchers have found that PCOS has a genetic component, different aspects of the syndrome being inherited by different family members as a result of faulty genes.[4] There may be male-pattern baldness in men (where the hairline recedes at the front and on the crown) and polycystic ovaries in women. As a result of their studies, experts believe that consideration of a woman's relatives can determine whether she will suffer from polycystic ovaries or not.

Of course, because ultrasound scanning was not readily available before the 1980s, a woman would have no way of knowing for sure whether her relatives had polycystic ovaries (or polycystic ovary syndrome) or not, although the symptoms are quite easy to define. It is possible to follow the trail through the generations, however, because certain illnesses – the long-term health risks of PCOS – may be seen in older relatives. These include conditions that occur in both sexes – adult-onset diabetes, high blood pressure and being overweight – while female relatives may have a history of infertility, hirsutism, menstrual problems and endometrial cancer.

It is not yet fully understood why one woman with polycystic ovaries has a regular monthly cycle and normal hormone levels, while another develops PCOS, but it is thought that genetic factors play a role. Each cell in the body has 23 pairs of chromosomes (46 altogether, including an X and a Y chromosome in men and two X chromosomes in women). Each chromosome contains thousands of genes, each of which controls the production of the proteins that instruct the body how to grow and function. Many diseases and medical conditions, including PCOS, occur because of faults in this genetic messenger system. Often a combination of genetic abnormalities is present, which is why different combinations of symptoms can manifest themselves in different people.

Studies have suggested that more than one gene is involved in the cause of PCOS. A 1997 study showed that, in PCOS, one of the faulty genes is involved in the first stage of testosterone production, which accounts for the raised levels of this hormone in the woman's bloodstream.[5] Experts believe that this gene probably interacts with other genes and with the environment to produce the final clinical picture. In another study, it was discovered that there is also a link between a specific variation in the insulin gene and the failure to ovulate in women with PCOS.[6] Research into the genetics of PCOS continues.

It is interesting that there also appear to be ethnic variations in the development of PCOS, with, for example, a higher preponderance among women from southern Asia than in white Caucasian women. Why this should be is not known.

Normal ovarian function

In PCOS, the hormonal household is in total disarray. However, in order to explain the many malfunctions, we need first of all to understand how the normal ovary works.

The ovaries are a pair of almond-shaped organs located deep within the female pelvis, behind the uterus (womb) and Fallopian tubes (see Figure 1, overleaf). The number of eggs that the ovaries carry is allotted before birth, when the ovaries are first formed. This means that new eggs are not produced, and so the eggs that a woman ovulates at the age of 40 are 40 years old. It appears that the better eggs are ovulated earlier in a woman's life and also that there is an increased risk of genetic or chromosomal abnormalities within the eggs as they grow older. This helps to explain the decline in fertility and the increased risk of miscarriage as women grow older, also the increased risk of chromosomal defects in children born to older mothers – Down's syndrome is just one example.

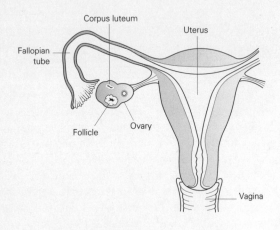

Figure 1 The female reproductive organs

When an egg is fertilized by the male sperm, an embryo results which should implant in the womb lining (endometrium) and ultimately become a baby. This cannot happen until a girl reaches puberty, until which time the eggs lie dormant. At the start of puberty, a substance called gonadotrophin releasing hormone (GnRH) is released by the hypothalamus (the body's hormonal control centre, located near the base of the brain) and secreted into the nearby pituitary gland (this gland is the command centre for the release of hormones from other glands, such as the ovaries, adrenal glands and thyroid). Here the release of luteinizing hormone (LH) and follicle stimulating hormone (FSH) are stimulated. As a result, the hypothalamus–pituitary–ovary pathway is fully awakened and the girl will start her periods (see Figure 2, opposite).

The normal menstrual cycle is often said to be 28 days in length, but in reality it can range from 23 to 35 days, as stated in Chapter 1. What is important is the regularity of the cycle, which should not vary by more than 1 or 2 days on either side of the average for the individual woman. The control of the cycle is determined by the release of GnRH from the hypothalamus and by feedback from the ovaries in the form of hormonal messages to the pituitary and hypothalamus. Stress and a change in body weight can upset the release of GnRH and disturb the monthly cycle.

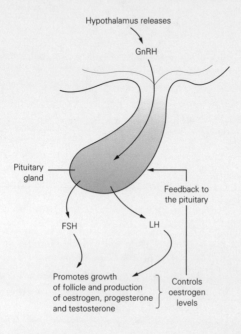

Hypothalamus releases

GnRH

Pituitary gland

Feedback to the pituitary

FSH   LH

Promotes growth
of follicle and production
of oestrogen, progesterone
and testosterone

Controls
oestrogen
levels

Figure 2 Multiple effects of the release of GnRH by the hypothalamus

The first half of the cycle – the 2 weeks before the egg is released from the ovarian follicle – is known as the follicular phase. It is this 'growing' phase of the cycle that varies between women, whereas the second half of the cycle, known as the luteal phase, is usually fairly constant in length (14 days in most women). The luteal phase occurs after the egg has been released and, generally, picked up into the Fallopian tube (ovulation). The follicle that has released the egg changes into a corpus luteum in the second half of the cycle, and it is this structure that produces progesterone after ovulation. Progesterone plays an important role in preparing the endometrium (womb lining) for the implantation of the embryo.

The follicular phase

During the follicular phase, follicle stimulating hormone (FSH) is released from the pituitary gland. This stimulates the follicles in the ovary to develop. One follicle in particular will quickly become dominant and so be the most likely to produce a mature egg. As soon as this occurs, the other eggs will stop ripening, allowing the dominant follicle to grow to a size of about 20 mm ($\frac{4}{5}$ inch). At the same time, LH is released, and together with FSH, the production of the hormones oestrogen and testosterone is promoted. Oestrogen production increases as the follicle continues to grow. It is normal for the ovary to also produce testosterone because oestrogen cannot be made without the presence of testosterone.

In the middle of the menstrual cycle, there is a final surge of LH. This causes the follicle to rupture and the egg to be released into one of the Fallopian tubes, from where it is transported towards the womb (uterus). Ovulation predictor kits that can be bought from chemist shops rely on the measurement of LH in the urine to detect the timing of ovulation.

The luteal phase

During the luteal phase of the cycle, the follicle changes in function to form the corpus luteum. This now produces progesterone, the main hormone for the remaining 2 weeks of the cycle. Progesterone ensures that the thickened womb lining secretes the nutrients that feed the egg if fertilization has occurred.

If fertilization has taken place as the egg travelled down the Fallopian tube, the egg continues to the womb where it is implanted in the womb lining. After implantation, the placenta of the developing pregnancy produces a hormone called human chorionic gonadotrophin (hCG) – the hormone that measures positive in a pregnancy test. This hormone stimulates the corpus luteum to continue to produce progesterone until about 12 weeks into the pregnancy. The embryo immediately begins to divide repeatedly until a foetus develops. The placenta secretes hormones for the duration of the pregnancy.

If fertilization has not taken place, however, production of progesterone and oestrogen ceases and the collapsed follicle (corpus luteum) begins to shrivel. The thickened womb lining then starts to break down and is shed as a menstrual period. The whole process of the menstrual cycle recommences at this point.

Abnormal ovarian function in PCOS

In PCOS, it appears that a malfunction within the hypothalamus–pituitary axis causes abnormal levels of hormones to be released. Levels of LH are often elevated, and it is the combination of this hormone and insulin that stimulates the production of testosterone by the ovaries. All women produce testosterone, which in normal circumstances is converted into oestrogen as the follicle grows, but in women with PCOS the levels of this hormone are higher than normal.

If a follicle fails to grow to maturity, as is often the case in PCOS, then the testosterone finds its way into the body's circulation and may have effects on the skin (acne, hair loss and unwanted hair growth). Testosterone may also be converted into oestrogen in the fat stores of the body, causing the woman to put on weight.

Oestrogen is required by the endometrium (womb lining) in order to help it to develop. Unfortunately, the abnormally high oestrogen levels in PCOS drive the thickening of the womb lining so much so that, ultimately, it may break down of its own accord, causing either a period or else spotting and bleeding in between periods.

The peppering of partially developed follicles around the periphery of the ovaries are the cysts that can be seen on ultrasound scans. Because of abnormal hormone levels, they have failed to develop into normal egg-producing follicles. However, even when a woman's cycle is irregular, a normal ovulation may occur from time to time, albeit in an unpredictable manner. Irregular cycles and problems with ovulation are the reason that some women with PCOS experience difficulty getting pregnant.

High levels of LH

As stated above, in the middle of the menstrual cycle, a final surge of LH is required to complete the development of the egg and allow it to be released from the follicle. However, when levels of LH are high throughout the cycle, as is often the case in PCOS, the development of the oocyte (egg cell) within the follicle may not take place properly. It is thought that if, unfortunately, ovulation occurs in the presence of a constantly high LH concentration throughout the follicular phase of the cycle, a time lapse between the ripening of the egg and its release may cause it to be prematurely aged, meaning either that it cannot be fertilized or that, if it is fertilized, it results in an abnormal embryo. The ultimate rejection of the embryo by the body gives us a reason for the occasional miscarriage seen in PCOS.

Raised levels of testosterone

When the ovaries themselves are not working as they should, their core and outer coating become thickened – and it is this thickened material that produces testosterone and other hormones that we normally associate with the male, and in higher amounts than is desirable. Testosterone is present in both sexes, but men produce ten times more than women. Excess production of this hormone in women is the cause of many PCOS symptoms, such as acne, excessive facial and body hair and the failure to ovulate (anovulation). Raised testosterone levels is the most common hormonal abnormality in PCOS, but not all sufferers are affected. On the other hand, some women are seriously affected.

It may be helpful to appreciate that the normal blood testosterone level in women is 0.5–3.5 nmol per litre (a tiny measure of a substance in solution); in men usually 15–30 nmol per litre. Women with PCOS usually have a testosterone level 2.5–5.0 nmol per litre. If the testosterone level is greater than 5 nmol per litre, it is important to look for other problems, such as testosterone-secreting tumours of the ovary or adrenal glands (which are very rare) and a condition called congenital adrenal hyperplasia, which is uncommon in the UK.

Testosterone is carried in the bloodstream by a protein called sex hormone binding globulin (SHBG). High insulin levels can suppress the production of SHBG so that the amount of active (or 'unbound') testosterone is elevated, which is why some women can have quite profound signs of testosterone excess in the presence of a normal blood concentration of the hormone. This is particularly the case in overweight women with high insulin levels.

The mild elevations in testosterone seen in women with PCOS can cause distressing symptoms (acne, hirsutism and alopecia – thinning of head hair), collectively known as androgenization or hyperandrogenism. However, testosterone levels in PCOS never get high enough to cause 'virilization', which is when the voice can become deeper, the breasts may shrink and the clitoris enlarge. If these effects occur, it is necessary to seek expert medical advice.

Insulin problems

In recent years it has become clear that there may be problems with insulin levels in PCOS and that, in fact, raised insulin levels in the blood appears to be one of the causes of the condition,[7] whether the woman is slim or overweight. Insulin is a hormone that is normally released from the pancreas after a meal. It allows the cells of the body to take up energy in the form of glucose, from which glycogen is released. Glucose is also stored as glycogen, by the liver (glycogen being a type of glucose that acts as a storage molecule and is used as a top-up when normal glucose levels have fallen). It is vital that glucose in the body is maintained at a stable level because brain function and normal body metabolism depend on it.

When glucose levels are not adequately controlled, diabetes is the inevitable result. High levels of blood glucose (hyperglycaemia) can cause excessive thirst, frequent urination and, ultimately, fainting and coma. Low levels of blood glucose (hypoglycaemia) can cause shakiness, dizziness, hunger, headaches, moodiness and confusion. If we eat more carbohydrate (glucose) in one meal than can be stored by the liver and the muscles, the excess is converted and stored in the fat cells.

Insulin resistance

Studies have found that, in PCOS, there is a resistance of the cells in the body to insulin. This means that the cells have difficulty converting glucose to energy. In an effort to compensate, the pancreas produces more insulin, which creates higher circulating levels of insulin than normal – a situation called hyperinsulinaemia. The result is often abnormal cholesterol and lipid levels, weight gain, irregular periods, higher levels of the androgens (the male hormones that all females have in low levels), infertility due to disturbance of ovulation and an increased likelihood of diabetes.

The excess insulin not only stimulates higher than normal androgen secretion (testosterone and so on) from the ovaries, it also appears to affect the normal development of the ovarian follicles. Because the incidence of diabetes in overweight women with PCOS is 11 per cent,[8] long-term screening of patients is advisable. Metformin, a diabetes treatment known as an insulin-sensitizing agent, can lower blood sugar levels and reduce high insulin levels.

Weight reduction may also achieve the same effect. (See Chapter 3 for more information on metformin.)

One study found insulin resistance in 30 per cent of slim women with PCOS, and in 75 per cent of overweight women with PCOS.[9] There was also a far higher percentage of women with a raised testosterone level in the latter group. This explains why overweight women with PCOS are more likely to suffer from hirsutism and infertility than slim women with PCOS.

Women with PCOS who have high levels of circulating insulin due to insulin resistance are at increased risk of developing diabetes during pregnancy. This is called gestational diabetes and can usually be managed by dietary modification. However, it sometimes requires drug therapy (including insulin injections). It is therefore recommended that overweight women lose weight before getting pregnant. Gestational diabetes generally disappears after pregnancy, but it signals an increased risk of developing diabetes again in later life.

Unfortunately, women with poorly controlled diabetes before they conceive run an increased risk of miscarriage and of difficulties during pregnancy and childbirth. They also have an increased risk of giving birth to babies with congenital malformations.

PCOS and being overweight

Being overweight may dramatically increase insulin levels and exaggerate all of the symptoms of PCOS. Oestrogen is made in the fat tissues and can lead to overgrowth of the lining of the endometrium (womb lining). If ovulation is not occurring and the endometrium becomes progressively thickened, the menstrual period, when it finally arrives, can be very heavy and painful. Furthermore, if there are excessively long gaps between periods, or if the periods are not happening at all, there is the risk of developing an abnormally thickened endometrium and, rarely, cancer of the womb. To prevent these things from happening, it is important to have a period once every 3 months, at the very least.

Losing weight can not only reduce the symptoms of PCOS, it can also normalize ovulation and therefore boost fertility. In a study of overweight women with PCOS who were not ovulating, 82 per cent began to ovulate after losing weight. In another study all but one woman with PCOS and fertility problems went on to conceive after losing weight. Another study examining the relationship between being overweight and fertility problems in PCOS found that once the women lost weight many of their hormonal problems resolved.

Weight loss can be difficult, but it will result in lower insulin levels and this in turn reduces testosterone production by the ovaries. It can be very difficult to sustain a healthy eating regime, and it is unfortunately quite common for women with PCOS to get into bad habits and develop disordered eating patterns, such as binge-eating and self-induced vomiting (known as bulimia nervosa). Indeed it has been suggested that nearly two-thirds of women with bulimia also have PCOS. If you have this kind of problem, see the Useful Addresses section on page 99 for details of eating disorders associations. It is important that bulimia be tackled correctly and sensitively or further problems may arise.

The long-term health risks of PCOS

The long-term health risks of PCOS are mainly related to the insulin problems and raised testosterone levels that generally play a part in the condition. High levels of insulin are associated with an increased risk of developing type 2 diabetes, which, if it develops, generally means strict diet control or possibly drug therapy. Between 25 and 35 per cent of overweight women with PCOS show signs of type 2 diabetes by their 30s and it becomes more common in women in their 40s and beyond. To prevent the later onset of diabetes, it is recommended that you follow a healthy eating plan and take regular exercise (see Chapter 5).

The hormone changes characteristic of PCOS increase the chance of later developing high blood pressure and high cholesterol levels, both of which can lead to a greater risk of heart disease. Again, a healthy eating plan and regular exercise can greatly reduce these risks.

As already mentioned, irregular or infrequent periods over a long length of time can lead to an increased risk of cancer of the endometrium (the womb lining). This risk is due to the high levels of oestrogen, which overstimulate the endometrium, causing it to continue to thicken. Normal shedding of the endometrium by way of regular periods effectively prevents endometrial cancer. If the endometrium appears thick on an ultrasound scan, or if irregular, prolonged bleeding occurs, a biopsy of the endometrium may be recommended. This can be done in the outpatient clinic or as a day-case surgical procedure. The womb lining is first inspected by a fine scope (a hysteroscope) and then a curettage or endometrial biopsy is performed.

For women with no periods at all, use of a low-dose contraceptive pill, or, for those who cannot take the pill, progesterone hormone treatment, can regulate periods and avoid the risk of endometrial cancer. As long as a menstrual period occurs at least once every 3 months, the risk of developing endometrial cancer is minimal.

As stated previously, irregular and heavy periods can occur as a result of problems with ovulation. While it would seem that restarting ovulation would be the best treatment, this is generally reserved for when a pregnancy is desired – ovarian stimulation drugs have potentially troublesome side-effects and need to be carefully monitored, making their long-term use inappropriate. However, the contraceptive pill and progesterone hormone treatment can stimulate menstruation (periods) without ovulation.

There does not appear to be a link between PCOS and ovarian cancer.

3

Getting Help from Your Doctor

If you think that you have PCOS, it is important to secure a diagnosis as early as possible. Without treatment of some kind – be it with conventional medicine or the holistic approach – long-term health problems become more of a risk.

Treatment appears to be effective in the majority of cases, and early diagnosis has the benefit of improving your long-term health outlook.

Preparing to see your doctor

If you are reading this book, you probably either suspect you have PCOS or already have a diagnosis of PCOS. For those who suspect, it is advised that you write down all your symptoms, even if some of them appear unrelated to PCOS – you may be suffering from another condition entirely. Abnormalities of the pituitary and adrenal glands can be associated with similar symptoms to those of PCOS. Obviously, if a tumour is detected immediate treatment is essential.

It is important to feel you that have the support of your doctor. If you are nervous about seeing your doctor on your own, it would probably be helpful to take a good friend or close family member with you to your appointment.

Note that teenagers who were prescribed the contraceptive pill to control heavy periods may only start displaying the symptoms of PCOS when they stop taking the pill, often several years after they were first prescribed it. For this reason, the diagnosis may be delayed for many years. In reality, the symptoms for which the pill was prescribed were the early manifestations of PCOS and when the pill is stopped the symptoms are unmasked once more.

It is likely to be helpful to make the following preparations for your visit to the surgery.

- Make a list of all the symptoms you have experienced in the past 4 weeks. These symptoms may include fatigue, depression, painful joints, bloating, tender breasts and mood swings. Write down a full and precise description of each symptom.

21

- If you are having periods, make a note of your monthly cycle, including heaviness of bleed, length of bleed and the average number of days from the start of one period to the start of the next one. Mention any spotting in between periods.
- If you are not having periods, make sure to write that down. Try to remember when your last period was and make a note of that too.
- Make a list of your other concerns – for example, excessive facial or body hair, weight gain, acne, hair loss and, if it is relevant, difficulty getting pregnant.
- Make a note of any questions you want to ask. Not only will this act as a memory prompt, it will also show the doctor that you feel the problem is serious.

At the consultation

Taking on board the following pointers should help you to get the best result from your doctor.

- Be as calm and relaxed as possible when talking to your doctor. Many doctors admit to feeling defensive and being less open-minded if the patient is in the least bit belligerent. In the same way, if you appear nervous, this can have the effect of making you appear unsure about your symptoms. Writing down everything beforehand should give you confidence.
- Tell your doctor that you have read about PCOS and suspect that this is your problem.
- Try to speak as clearly and slowly as is reasonable, so that your doctor misses nothing.
- Each time your doctor asks you a question, be sure you have understood before making your reply.
- You may be told you are being sent for tests, which is the result you want. If the doctor doesn't mention tests, make the suggestion yourself. In the unlikely event that your doctor doesn't think tests are required, be sure to ask what other causes there might be for your symptoms. Remember that if you are unhappy with your doctor's conclusions you are entitled to a second opinion.

What tests am I likely to have?

PCOS can easily be determined by blood tests and an ultrasound scan.

Blood tests

Blood tests help to rule out similar conditions and can confirm a diagnosis of PCOS. Your doctor will probably arrange for blood to be taken during days 1–3 of your menstrual period, if you are having periods. If you are not, blood can be taken at any time, but the test may need to be repeated.

Blood samples may be used for the following tests.

- Androgen levels: although not all women with PCOS have raised testosterone and androstenedione – the androgen hormones – these abnormalities are very common in PCOS.
- LH, which stimulates the ovary to produce testosterone. Again, although high levels of LH are often seen in PCOS, there are many exceptions. Normal levels should not rule out a diagnosis. This test is best carried out on day 1–3 of a menstrual bleed. If periods are absent or infrequent, then a random sample can be taken.
- FSH: again this test should be taken on day 1–3 of a menstrual bleed, but it can be done randomly where periods are absent or irregular. FSH is quite a good predictor of the fertility potential of the ovaries.
- SHBG, levels of which may be low in PCOS.
- Insulin: levels of insulin in the blood are not usually measured since the test is complicated and therefore only performed as part of research. However, insulin resistance can be determined by performing a glucose tolerance test. The glucose tolerance test should be carried out if the woman is overweight (body mass index more than 30 kg/m^2). The test is performed on an empty stomach after an overnight fast. A sugary drink is given and blood taken at the start and again after 2 hours. As south Asian women with PCOS are more likely to develop insulin resistance at a lower weight than seen in the female Caucasian population, a glucose tolerance test is advised in these women if the body mass index is more than 25 kg/m^2.
- Thyroid function: as some of the symptoms of PCOS are similar to those of thyroid malfunction, this test is also necessary.

- Prolactin levels: prolactin is a hormone that, when elevated, can be associated with irregular or absent periods, and its levels should therefore be checked.
- Full blood count, which will show whether you have adequate red blood cells, whose role is to carry oxygen around your body. If not, the result is often fatigue and anaemia.

If blood tests suggest that you have PCOS, your GP or specialist may send you for an ultrasound scan.

Ultrasound scan

Ultrasound scans are now often carried out at local medical centres. Alternatively, you may be sent to your nearest hospital. As a full bladder makes the reading clearer, those undergoing an external scan will be asked to drink up to 2 litres of water beforehand. A small amount of clear gel is placed on the lower abdomen, and the probe is then moved around the surface area. Ultrasound waves are bounced off the ovaries to create a picture. A woman with PCOS will have ovaries that show lots of tiny cysts around the edge of the ovary, in a 'pearl necklace' effect. These are the partially developed eggs that were not released from the follicles into the Fallopian tubes.

Women undergoing an internal scan – where a small ultrasound probe is placed just inside the vagina – do not need a full bladder before the scan. An internal scan gives a clearer view of the ovaries and pelvic organs and should not cause pain.

If the endometrium is seen to be thicker than 15 mm ($\frac{3}{5}$ inch) on the scan, a period may be induced by specific medication, usually a short course of progestogen tablets.

What happens after the diagnosis?

Once your doctor has concluded that your problem is indeed PCOS, there are several possible courses of action. Conventional medical treatment – using drug therapy – is generally the first step in treating the symptoms, but if you wish to attempt to tackle the underlying causes of the disorder, you could also try the holistic approach, as discussed in the next chapter. Most doctors are pleased to hear that their patient is, as an adjunct to drug therapy, making efforts to help herself. However, the medications offered generally give more immediate results and may be used until such a time as holistic treatments take effect. For women who find holistic treatments difficult to maintain or for whom the effect is less than that desired, medications may be the only effective way forward.

Because many of the drugs that treat the symptoms of PCOS prevent pregnancy, your doctor will, first of all, want to know whether you are trying to get pregnant. There are some therapies that should not be taken while you are trying to conceive (for example, tetracyclines, spironolactone, flutamide, finasteride) and reliable contraception will therefore be advised. Remember that even if you are not having periods you may ovulate without warning from time to time. If you do not wish to conceive you must *always* use reliable contraception. (Women with infrequent periods and no wish for a pregnancy sometimes get pregnant, not realizing until it is too late to have the pregnancy terminated.)

Try not to feel daunted by the large number of medications presented in this book – it means only that there is a great deal of help available. It also means that if one type of drug is not suitable for whatever reason, there is generally an equally effective alternative.

Medications that regulate your periods

If you do not wish to get pregnant, a low dose of the oral contraceptive pill can regulate your monthly menstrual cycle. Any combined oral contraceptive pill (COCP) can achieve this. All COCPs can cause an elevation in SHBG levels and also suppress testosterone production by the ovaries and so improve the symptoms of hyperandrogenism – the mild elevations of testosterone seen in PCOS. Sometimes Dianette or Yasmin are prescribed, because, as well as bringing the cycle to a normal 28 days and making blood loss more normal, they also contain progestogens, the hormones that help to counteract the effects of androgens (testosterone and so on). Dianette contains cyproterone acetate, an anti-androgen that can improve acne and hirsutism; Yasmin contains drosperinone, which is a derivative of spironolactone (the main anti-androgen used in the USA).

Unfortunately, the pill is known to exacerbate the problem of insulin resistance – and there are many possible side-effects linked with the pill. Those related to Dianette include leg pains and cramps, depression, enlargement of the breasts, fluid retention, weight gain, headaches, nausea, loss of libido, and vaginal discharge. Women with diabetes, asthma, varicose veins or hypertension (high blood pressure) should not take this drug since it can worsen the condition. Dianette may very occasionally affect the liver, and therefore liver function, by way of a blood test, should be assessed before Dianette is started and again after 6 months of therapy. Like all COCPs, Dianette has been associated with an increased risk of venous thromboembolism, examples of which are deep vein thrombosis, pulmonary embolism and stroke. The risks may be higher with Dianette than with lower dose COCPs, so it is generally recommended to switch from Dianette to a lower-dose preparation once symptoms of PCOS are well controlled. This may be after about 6 months.

Many women report that the pill masks their PCOS symptoms while they are using it but that when they stop taking it, their symptoms worsen. Indeed, this is precisely how the pill is designed to work. However, all drugs may have adverse effects. It is generally a matter of looking at the benefits and weighing up whether they are worth those effects. Each case is highly individual and some will find more benefit than others.

An alternative to the COCP is one of the progestogen-only preparations, which can induce regular withdrawal bleeds if taken on a cyclical basis (for example for 12 days every 1–3 months to induce a bleed). Such preparations include medroxyprogesterone acetate (Provera) and dydrogesterone (Duphaston). The side-effects linked with these drugs are probably worse than those of the COCP and include weight gain, fluid retention, abnormal production of breast milk, gastrointestinal upset, breast pain and acne. Obviously, some of these possible effects, if they arise, are counter-productive to women with PCOS, and alternative medications may have to be tried. As women with PCOS are thought to be at increased risk of later developing heart disease, a COCP that contains agents that reduce the effects of dietary fats could be used. Ask your GP or specialist about this.

Any irregular bleeding while you are taking hormone-based medications should be checked by your doctor, who may advise an ultrasound scan or curettage surgery. A cervical (Pap) smear should be taken at least once every 3 years in all sexually active women.

As an alternative to medications, a progestogen-releasing intra-uterine coil (Mirena) may be offered. This type of coil can effectively prevent the abnormal build-up of the endometrium (womb lining). The one main side-effect can be unpredictable light bleeding or discharge, and occasionally the periods may stop altogether. However, because this occurs when the endometrium has become thin, it is safe.

Medications that treat hirsutism and acne

Hirsutism and acne are the result of elevated levels of testosterone in the female body, testosterone levels being dictated by the amount of SHBG in the blood. High levels of insulin lower the production of SHBG from the liver and so increase the levels of active (free) testosterone.

Your specialist may use a standardized scoring system such as the modified Ferriman and Gallwey score to evaluate the degree of hirsutism before and during drug therapy. The Ferriman and Gallwey score enables a record to be kept of the amount of unwanted hair covering the different parts of the body. It is, of course, difficult to make such an assessment if other methods (such as shaving, waxing, electrolysis or laser) are being used to deal with the unwanted hair.

When Dianette or Yasmin fail to tackle the problem of acne and hirsutism sufficiently, a preparation called Androcur may be prescribed in addition – this formulation contains cyproterone acetate in a higher dose than found in Dianette (50 mg daily rather than 2 mg). However, cyproterone acetate must be taken with adequate contraception, since foetal abnormality can occur if the drug is used in early pregnancy. Cyproterone acetate should be taken for the first 10 days of a cycle alongside the contraceptive pill for the first 21 days. Within a gap of 7 days, menstruation should occur and the regimen is repeated. The effect on acne is usually seen within a couple of months; however, the effect on hirsutism and alopecia (hair loss) may take much longer. As cyproterone can have a detrimental affect on the liver, liver function should be regularly checked, by way of a blood test, during treatment.

Spironolactone is another option for treating stubborn acne and hirsutism, but this drug frequently causes erratic periods and is often given with a low-dose contraceptive pill. Spironolactone is a mild diuretic (it reduces water retention and lowers blood pressure in those with elevated blood pressure) and is commonly used when it is unsafe to use the COCP – for example, in cases of extreme obesity, in smokers over the age of 35, or in high blood pressure.

Other medications aimed particularly at hirsutism include flutamide and finasteride – and again reliable contraception is essential. The side-effects of these anti-androgens include tiredness, mood changes and reduced sex drive. As with other anti-androgens, flutamide can impair liver function, so tests should be carried out every 6 months.

Owing to the slow rate of hair growth, all hirsutism treatments must be continued for up to 18 months before a response may be seen. During that time, depilatory creams, electrolysis, laser, bleaching, waxing and shaving could be used.

Medications that treat obesity

There are now medications that inhibit the absorption of fat from the diet. However, since they inhibit good fats as well as bad fats, they should be used only when all else has failed and only in the short term to start the process of weight reduction. There is no substitute for a healthy weight-loss plan. (For more information on diet, see Chapter 5.)

Medications that treat insulin resistance

The first line of attack regarding insulin resistance is weight loss. The next step is to consider a drug called metformin (also known as Glucophage) – an 'anti-diabetic' drug that is often used to treat non-insulin-dependent (or type 2) diabetes. For women with PCOS, this medication has been shown to lower levels of insulin, testosterone and LH and to raise levels of SHBG.[10] As a result, menstruation can often be regulated, ovulation may occur, and the symptoms of androgen excess (hirsutism, acne etc.) may decline.[11]

Another pleasing effect when metformin is combined with a healthy diet and exercise can be weight loss in those who were overweight. In a 1998 study, metformin was shown to improve the menstrual pattern with minimal endocrine and metabolic effects in

PCOS.[12] All in all, metformin has benefits for both short-term and long-term health. Not all women lose weight while taking metformin, however, and again there is no substitute for a healthy diet and exercise. Note that this drug is not yet a licensed treatment of PCOS and can be prescribed for PCOS only by an endocrinologist or specialist in reproductive medicine. Metformin therapy may be continued in the long term, but it should, for safety, be stopped during pregnancy (although detrimental effects on either pregnancy or the foetus have not been reported).

When starting to take metformin, patients will often experience an upset stomach, diarrhoea and flatulence. These problems usually resolve after the first week or two and they can be minimized by taking the drug with a meal and by starting on a low dosage. It is recommended that patients start with one 500 mg pill daily the first week and increase this to twice a day during the second week. If stomach upsets are minimal after the second week, the dose can be raised to 850 mg twice daily. Other side-effects linked with this drug are various endocrine disorders (hormonal problems), repeated infections, agitation, stress, allergic reaction and skin rashes.

People taking metformin should discontinue the medication immediately if shortness of breath, severe muscle weakness or chest pain is experienced. It should also be stopped 48 hours before surgery and 48 hours before an X-ray study in which dye is administered (such as an intravenous pyelogram). It should not be taken by people who use alcohol excessively.

You will be asked to return to your doctor 3 months after starting metformin. If you have successfully ovulated and wish to conceive, therapy will continue for another 3 months to see if you can get pregnant. As stated, this medication should be stopped if pregnancy occurs.

Your doctor may wish to prescribe pioglitazone (also known as Actos) or rosiglitazone (also known as Avandia), or both, either in place of metformin or to work alongside it as a combination therapy. These medications have been known to reverse the endocrine abnormalities seen in PCOS within 2 or 3 months. They can result in diminished facial or body hair, regulation of the menstrual cycle, normalization of high blood pressure, decreased hair loss from the head, weight loss and improvement in fertility. Some women have even conceived in their first ovulatory cycle after taking these medications. Studies have shown that by 6 months over 90 per cent of women treated with these insulin-lowering agents may resume regular periods.

Women taking pioglitazone or rosiglitazone are seen at 2-monthly intervals for monitoring of their liver function. Ovulation is monitored and, after 4 months, laboratory tests re-evaluated. The level of C-peptide – and insulin secretion – may also be tested.

If therapy is not proving successful the dose of drugs may be increased or combinations prescribed.

The few studies conducted into the use of insulin-sensitizing drugs as a treatment of PCOS suggest that they may well be beneficial. They appear to help to regulate menstruation and help to facilitate ovulation. Sometimes there is an improvement in weight and blood cholesterol levels. Weight reduction is a more variable finding. One study looking at ovulation in particular found that it occurred in 34 per cent of the women who were taking metformin.[13] When metformin was combined with a drug called clomiphene citrate (also known as Clomid; see Chapter 4 for more information about clomiphene citrate), 90 per cent of women ovulated compared with 8 per cent of those who received only clomiphene citrate. These study groups were made up of overweight women with PCOS. Whether the same results would be seen in women of normal weight has not yet been established.

It is important to note that pioglitazone and rosiglitazone carry the same possible side-effects as metformin. The side-effects linked to clomiphene citrate include hot flushes, abdominal discomfort, blurred vision and enlargement of the ovaries.

4

Getting Pregnant

As we have seen, several types of medication are capable of kick-starting normal ovarian function and may therefore help you to achieve a pregnancy. As well as detailing the most effective of those medications, this chapter discusses some of the medical procedures involved in conception. (See Chapter 7 for help with the emotional repercussions that may arise during this difficult time.)

Preparing to get pregnant

General health measures are important when trying to conceive, and a healthy diet is essential (see Chapter 5). Smoking can not only be harmful to your health, it also reduces your chances of having a successful pregnancy. It is therefore important not to smoke if you are trying for a baby. In addition to reducing fertility, smoking is associated with the earlier onset of the menopause and an increased risk of miscarriage, stillbirth and cot death.

It is also sensible to abstain from alcohol, which is believed to have a significant effect on both female and male fertility.

Remember that if you are wishing to conceive you should be taking 0.4 mg folic acid daily. This has been shown to reduce the incidence of some developmental anomalies in the baby, such as spina bifida.

Weight reduction in overweight women with PCOS

It is estimated that 85 per cent of women with ovulatory difficulties suffer from PCOS. Because the syndrome is more common in overweight women, weight reduction should be your first step – this may even start spontaneous ovulation. The amount of weight loss necessary is less than you might think, for a reduction of only 5 per cent of a sufferer's current weight is associated with an increased number of ovulatory cycles. Furthermore, even if spontaneous ovulation does not occur there is an increased chance of responding to the drugs that promote ovulation if you can lose weight. It is therefore sensible that you should immediately start following a healthy eating plan (see Chapter 5). This will not only benefit a pregnancy and the child at the end of it, but it will also help to reduce the symptoms of your PCOS.

Initial investigations

If you have been diagnosed with PCOS and the time is right for you and your partner to start trying for a family you should go to your doctor straight away and ask to be referred to your local specialist fertility clinic. As the referral may take a few months to come through, your own GP may initiate some investigations that will help to speed things up.

Initial investigations include checking that you are immune to rubella (German measles) before you conceive. Hormone levels (FSH, LH, testosterone, thyroid function and prolactin) will be checked usually on days 1–3 of the cycle, or at random if you do not have a cycle. Progesterone will be checked approximately 7 days before your expected period (day 21 of a 28-day cycle), although there is little point in measuring progesterone if your periods are very irregular. At some stage your partner should provide a semen sample for analysis too.

Checking ovulation

Many women like to use home predictor kits to check whether ovulation is occurring. It is our advice that they are generally not worthwhile since they can be expensive and do not really help if your cycle is erratic. If, on the other hand, your cycle is regular then you *are* ovulating and there is no need to do your own tests. The sort of tests we are referring to most commonly measure LH in the urine. LH is the hormone that is released in a surge about 40 hours before ovulation takes place. Some women with PCOS have high circulating levels of LH throughout their cycle, causing the urine to test falsely positive when a surge is not actually happening.

As the body's temperature rises by 0.2–0.5°C (0.4–0.9°F) shortly after ovulation (an effect of progesterone), temperature testing used to be popular. However, because this method is not very reliable and causes stress, it is no longer recommended.

When to make love

Couples wishing to conceive worry about when to make love and often think it is best to delay having intercourse until around the time of ovulation. While it is, of course, true that sperm need to be present in the Fallopian tubes when the egg is released, it is actually not good to have long gaps between ejaculations. This is because sperm, unlike eggs, is manufactured daily and stored before release – and the longer that sperm is stored the older it gets. The sperm count may slowly increase, but sperm function tends to decline.

The optimum time between ejaculations is 2–3 days, so it is advisable to try to make love at least every 3 days in the first half of the cycle and perhaps a little more frequently (every 1–2 days) around the time of anticipated ovulation. If you are having regular periods (that is, with a cycle length of between 21 and 35 days but not varying by more than 2–3 days on either side of the average length each month) then you are likely to be ovulating 14 days before your period is due. Remember that it is the second half of the cycle, after ovulation, that is the most constant in terms of length.

At the fertility clinic

When you attend the fertility clinic you will be examined, swabs may be taken from the cervix to rule out the presence of infection and you will be advised to have a test to check that your Fallopian tubes are open.

Checking the Fallopian tubes

There are two ways of checking the Fallopian tubes. The simplest way is via an X-ray called a hysterosalpingogram (HSG), which is performed in the X-ray department within 10 days of either a natural or artificially induced period (to rule out the risk of a pregnancy). X-ray dye is gently injected through the cervix and X-ray pictures taken to provide an outline of the inside of the womb and also of the Fallopian tubes.

If any abnormalities appear on the HSG, or if you have a history of gynaecological problems, you may be advised to undergo a laparoscopy. This is an operative procedure performed under general anaesthetic in which a scope is passed through a small incision just below the umbilicus (belly button). Through the scope it is possible for the surgeon to see all the pelvic structures and to assess the womb, Fallopian tubes and ovaries. It should be possible to deal with simple problems at the time of the initial laparoscopy – such as adhesions (scar tissue) around the ovaries and tubes from previous infection or endometriosis. Sometimes it is necessary to perform more extensive surgery at a later date.

Stimulating ovulation

For induction of ovulation to be successful it is important that the Fallopian tubes and pelvic organs should be healthy and that sperm function should be normal. If significant problems are detected during these baseline investigations, it may be necessary to proceed straight to *in vitro* fertilization (IVF) (see below).

Before induction of ovulation, you may also be advised to have a glucose tolerance test (see Chapter 3). If you are overweight you may be referred to a dietician and you may also be advised to take metformin (see Chapter 3). The most commonly used drug to stimulate ovulation is clomiphene citrate (also known as Clomid), an anti-oestrogen hormonal preparation that stimulates the release of FSH by the pituitary gland. Clomiphene citrate should be taken in the early days of the cycle (usually days 2–6). If you are not having regular periods you may be given a short course of a progestogen, such as medroxyprogesterone acetate, in order to induce an artificial bleed – after first having a pregnancy test to ensure that you are not pregnant.

Clomiphene citrate achieves ovulation in about 80 per cent of women but, as with all fertility therapies, pregnancy does not necessarily occur straight away. It is important to appreciate that, even for optimally fertile couples in their mid-20s, the best chance of a spontaneous pregnancy in 1 month is about 25 per cent; after 6 months the chance has risen to about 60 per cent. After 1 year approximately 85 per cent will have conceived. Fertility therapies rarely better this natural, cumulative chance of conception over time; moreover, these therapies are usually given to couples who are in an older age group and who therefore have an age-related reduced chance of pregnancy.

With clomiphene citrate the chance of conception is about 40–50 per cent after 6 months, rising slowly thereafter. The risk of multiple pregnancy is about 10 per cent. The starting dose is 50 mg a day and this may be increased to 100 mg if the lower dose does not work. Once regular ovulation is being achieved the therapy may be continued for 6 months initially, then reviewed and sometimes continued, but not for more than 9–12 months.

Clomiphene citrate therapy must be monitored by regular ultrasound scan in order to:

- ensure that a response is occurring,
- ensure that the timing of intercourse coincides with ovulation,
- help to reduce the risk of multiple pregnancy.

This type of therapy should generally be administered from and monitored by a fertility clinic with appropriate facilities for ultrasound monitoring.

An alternative to clomiphene citrate is tamoxifen, which works in the same way. The side-effects of both include hot flushes, abdominal discomfort and blurred vision. In the short term, reversible hair loss is occasionally experienced.

If ovulation does not occur in response to clomiphene citrate, then the options are either gonadotrophin therapy or laparoscopic ovarian diathermy. If, on the other hand, ovulation occurs but a pregnancy does not result the next step is usually to move on to assisted conception, in the form of IVF.

Gonadotrophin therapy involves the daily injection of hormone preparations containing FSH. FSH can be purified from the urine of post-menopausal women, where it is found in high concentration along with LH. The two together constitute human menopausal gonadotrophin (hMG), which is available these days in a number of different formulations. An alternative is genetically engineered (or 'recombinant') FSH. The injections are usually given just under the skin (subcutaneously) and you can be taught how to administer them yourself. Some preparations require deeper, intramuscular injections. The starting dose is usually 50–75 units a day, and this may be increased or decreased depending on the response.

Gonadotrophin therapy requires very careful monitoring because the numerous follicles within the polycystic ovary are sensitive to stimulation. Once the threshold dose has been reached, the ovaries may almost explode into action producing far more growing follicles than the single one needed to produce the required egg. Ultrasound monitoring is usually commenced after 1 week of injections and scans are then performed every 2–3 days until the largest follicle has reached a size of 17–18 mm (about $\frac{3}{4}$ inch). An injection of human chorionic gonadotrophin (hCG) is then given to trigger the release of the egg. The hCG injection should be withheld if there are three or more follicles larger than 14 mm (about $\frac{1}{2}$ inch) because of the risk of multiple pregnancy.

In one study, the number of pregnancies achieved after ovarian stimulation with gonadotrophins reached 62 per cent after 6 months and 73 per cent after 12 months.[14] In the same study, live births reached 54 per cent after 6 months and 62 per cent after 12 months.

Women with PCOS are also at risk of developing a rare but serious condition called ovarian hyperstimulation syndrome, in which too many follicles are stimulated. Because this may result in abdominal distension, discomfort, nausea, vomiting and sometimes difficulty breathing, close monitoring is essential and sometimes hospital admission is required.

As stated above, an alternative to gonadotrophin is laparoscopic ovarian diathermy (LOD), also known as 'ovarian drilling'. This procedure is performed under general anaesthesia in a way similar to the laparoscopic assessment of the pelvis (see above). The aim is to cause four small burns on each ovary as, somewhat surprisingly, this appears to kick-start the ovary into action. If ovulation fails to occur straight away the ovaries often become more receptive to clomiphene citrate or gonadotrophin therapy. The operation of LOD has taken the place of 'wedge resection', which was a more major operation in which a large part of the ovary was removed in order to make it a more normal size. The problem with that was the loss of eggs and the potential for significant scarring around the ovaries and Fallopian tubes. LOD, however, carries all the inherent risks of a surgical operation.

The success rates of gonadotrophin therapy are better after six cycles than at six months after LOD. By 12 months, however, the results are similar. The greatest success rates of LOD are in women with a shorter length of infertility (less than 3 years) and those with an elevated level of LH. The advantages of LOD include the reduced risk of multiple pregnancy and the reduced need for monitoring. In practical terms LOD is usually best for women who find it difficult to attend the clinic for regular and frequent scans and for those who persistently over-respond to gonadotrophin therapy.[15]

IVF

When ovarian stimulation is unsuccessful, many women resort to IVF. Success rates here depend very much on individual characteristics such as age, length of infertility and body weight. Because ovarian stimulation and IVF are less successful if a woman is very overweight, most clinics encourage weight loss before the commencement of therapy. Metformin (see Chapter 3) may be of benefit together with fertility treatments. Much research is currently under way to assess the true role of IVF in PCOS.

The process of IVF involves a more complex regimen of drug therapy than is the case in straightforward induction of ovulation. Each clinic varies slightly in its protocols, but you will certainly be given detailed information and an opportunity to talk things through both with a doctor and with a counsellor. Drugs may be prescribed before ovarian stimulation is started, and these sometimes include the combined oral contraceptive pill to regulate the cycle, GnRH (see page 12), drugs such as buserelin and nafarelin to switch off the pituitary gland, and then FSH or hMG to stimulate the ovaries.

Ovarian stimulation takes on average 9–10 days and then an hCG injection is given at night when the follicles have reached the prerequisite size. The egg collection is then performed 36 hours later, while the woman is mildly sedated. A needle is guided through the vagina under ultrasound vision into the ovaries to draw out the eggs (oocytes) from the follicles. The eggs are next placed in an incubator in the laboratory with sperm produced that day. If there is a problem with the sperm then one sperm may be injected into each egg – a procedure called intercytoplasmic sperm injection. After 2 days in the incubator, two embryos are transferred into the uterus (womb) through the cervix in a procedure that is rather like having a smear test. Progesterone pessaries are then usually taken daily until the results of a pregnancy test are known two weeks later.

Extensive research has shown that the drugs used during IVF appear to be safe, although some women may experience side-effects, such as headaches, hot flushes, mood swings, tender breasts and a sore abdomen. There is also a risk of ovarian hyperstimulation syndrome (see above). We advise that you use all the stress management techniques available to you during this difficult time.

In cases where the administered hormones do not produce the required result, it may be possible to alter the dosages and try again during the next menstrual cycle. The success rate of IVF is about 25–30 per cent per cycle, depending on a number of factors. The chances of a healthy birth increase to 60 per cent after six completed cycles of treatment. Each time pregnancy fails to occur, there are generally feelings of intense disappointment, grief and anger and a sense of failure. Most clinics have a trained counsellor on hand, who will offer to discuss your feelings with you after each failed attempt.

The counsellor will realize that this is a difficult time for both partners and that it is likely to be putting enormous strain on the relationship (see Chapter 7 for information on emotional support).

A number of factors are now recognized as influencing the chance of achieving a pregnancy, and after one cycle of treatment it may become obvious that an alternative treatment is more suitable in your situation.

5

Helping Yourself

There is no doubt that medications can play an important role in controlling the symptoms of PCOS and that they can be invaluable in achieving a pregnancy. However, PCOS is a lifelong condition that invariably responds better when also managed by the sufferer. The long-term health risks are often minimized when the person takes her health into her own hands.

Improving your diet

It is now clear that the symptoms of PCOS can be exacerbated by stress, a poor diet and environmental toxins. Some experts believe that, in women who are genetically predisposed to developing the condition, a high fat diet with lots of stimulants (such as caffeine, sugar and alcohol) and exposure to certain environmental chemicals can actually trigger it. However, there is evidence that cutting down on saturated fats and stimulants can reduce the symptoms.

After seeing your doctor, making dietary improvements should, ideally, be the second step in your journey towards better health. Eating more healthily may not be a cure, but it can help to reduce the symptoms of PCOS. It can also help to minimize the long-term health risks associated with the condition.

People's diets have become very poor over the years. Crop production is now loaded with chemicals, and more chemicals are then added to allow foods to travel long distances and to withstand a long shelf-life. Added chemicals not only keep food looking fresh, they are intended to enhance the flavour. However, foods that have been refined and processed in this way hold little nutritional value and the chemical content is known to be harmful to health.[16] As a consequence, we constantly ingest low levels of toxins, which are then likely to upset the hormone levels within the body. As hormone levels in PCOS are already abnormal, further disturbance may only exacerbate the situation.

The following points outline current food habits.

- We eat food that has been sprayed many times with chemical pesticides, herbicides and fungicides. These poisons kill essential soil microbes that would otherwise help plants to absorb nutrient-rich minerals such as zinc, copper, magnesium and manganese, which are essential to good health.
- We eat food grown on land that has been artificially fertilized with nitrogen, potassium and phosphorus instead of manure or compost. Although artificial fertilizers stimulate plant growth, their use has greatly reduced the mineral content of soil. It also causes an imbalance in our hormone levels. Organically grown foods may be a little more expensive, but they are toxin-free and they do taste good.
- Plant foods are then artificially ripened, stored and processed. Unfortunately, the refining and storage process robs food of the majority of its fibre and nutrients. Most of the precious B vitamins and vitamin E are lost in the processing and bleaching of wheat and flour, leaving it valueless and literally poisonous to the body. Similarly, all other cereals, fruits and vegetables lose much of their nutrients and vitamin C during processing.
- We eat the tasty parts of the food only, disposing of the rest. For example, wheat husks and wheatgerm – the most nutritious parts of the plant – are removed before the remaining cereal is processed into white flour. 'Whole' foods contain fibre and so aid the removal of waste materials from the bowel. They are vital to good bowel health.

Cutting out food additives

Cutting out additives such as food colourings, preservatives and flavourings (usually listed on the tin or packet as 'E numbers') should ensure that the toxicity that interferes with our hormone levels is reduced, and it can even help to rebalance the body.

Unfortunately, the majority of the foods on our supermarket shelves have undergone some degree of chemical refinement or alteration. The additives that cause most harm are monosodium glutamate (MSG), artificial colourings, butylated hydroxyanisole (BHA), butylated hydroxytoluene (BHT), sorbate, sulphites and aspartame.

Contrary to popular belief, aspartame will not help you to lose weight. It is known to trigger a craving for carbohydrate and will cause you to put on weight. At a recent World Environment Conference, one doctor revealed that when he got people off aspartame, their average weight loss was 8.5 kg (19 lb) per person. Aspartame is commonly found in foods described as 'low sugar', 'sugar free', or 'diet . . .'.

What should women with PCOS eat?

Eating a well-balanced, organic, wholefood diet can be of great benefit to women with PCOS. It may be difficult, at first, to make the recommended changes, but the benefit to your overall health will make the effort worthwhile. However, if you find you are unable to make great changes, don't feel guilty or despondent. Small changes are better than no change at all. They will make a difference.

Reducing sugar and refined carbohydrates

Our diets today are often high in sugar and refined carbohydrates (which are found in biscuits, cakes, pastries and so on). Unfortunately, refined carbohydrates cause a rapid rise in blood glucose levels. When we consistently consume high levels of sugar and refined carbohydrates, our bodies make an excess of insulin, which, as we have seen, can be detrimental to women with PCOS, causing an increase in weight and exacerbating the symptoms. Furthermore, this type of food holds little nutritional value, and it uses a great deal of energy in its digestion, absorption and elimination.

Sugar – which has been dubbed 'the scourge of the age' – contains no nutritional value at all. In fact, sugar consumption has been linked with many disorders, from diabetes to heart disease and cancer. You probably know that sugar converts into energy. What you may not know is that we can actually obtain all the sugars and energy we need from fruit and complex (unrefined) carbohydrates (in grains and lentils, for example). Unrefined carbohydrates are converted into sugar in the body as nature intended.

Reducing salt

Salt is commonly used as a preservative and is added to most processed, pre-packaged foods – breakfast cereals, for example, are high in salt. As a result, people who eat a lot of processed foods may

41

be consuming more salt than they realize, especially when the salt used in cooking and at the table is also taken into account. However, wholefoods actually contain salt (sodium) and potassium in just the right balance for our bodies. Extra salt upsets this happy balance and can lead to a variety of problems. Try using herbs and spices (in moderation) for flavouring. Sea salt contains more minerals than ordinary salt, but it is still salt – so use it sparingly.

Reducing red meat and dairy produce

Saturated fats from dairy produce and red meat are recommended only in moderation in PCOS since they can stimulate the body to produce too much oestrogen and prostaglandins, and a woman with PCOS has an excess of these hormones already. In addition, consumption of red meat slows down the waste elimination process, causing the body to reabsorb oestrogen that has become compacted in the bowel.

White meat and fish – particularly oily fish such as herring, mackerel, sardines and tuna – are good sources of protein and oils, but a piece no larger than the palm of your hand should be eaten. Try to ensure that you buy only organic meat – that is, from animals reared without the use of antibiotics, anabolic steroids, chemical pesticides and so on.

Reducing caffeine products

Caffeine products, which include coffee, tea, cocoa, cola drinks and chocolate, cause stress to the adrenal glands. They are also toxic to the liver and can reduce the body's ability to absorb vitamins and minerals. If caffeine is consumed regularly in fairly high quantities, it is likely to give rise to chronic anxiety, the symptoms of which are agitation, palpitations, headaches, indigestion, panic, insomnia and hyperventilation. More than two cups of coffee a day has been linked to the development of endometriosis.[17] The best advice is to remove caffeine products from your diet.

Unfortunately, the addictiveness of caffeine makes reduction far from easy, and withdrawal symptoms can take the form of splitting headaches, fatigue, depression, poor concentration and muscle pains. It is no wonder that people can feel terrible until they have had their first dose of caffeine in the morning and that they can't seem to function properly without regular doses throughout the day! Fortunately, caffeine is quickly 'washed out' of the system – and it is possible to minimize withdrawal symptoms by reducing your intake over several weeks.

A problem for many is finding an acceptable alternative. Coffee, tea, cocoa and cola drinks can be replaced by fruit and vegetable juices, herbal teas – green tea is very good, as is rooibosch (redbush) tea. They are both low in tannin and high in antioxidants. A variety of grain coffee substitutes may also be purchased from health-food shops. As many decaffeinated products are processed with the use of chemicals, they are not a good choice.

Carob, which is similar to the cocoa bean, is a healthy, caffeine-free alternative to cocoa and chocolate. It contains less fat and is naturally sweet, unlike the cocoa bean which is bitter and needs sweetening. Many people find carob bars an enjoyable replacement for chocolate bars and other confectionery. It is also available in powder form for use in baking and in drinks.

Dietary fats

Fats (fatty acids) are the most concentrated sources of energy in our diet, 1 g of fat providing the body with 9 calories of energy.

However, as you are probably aware, some types of fat are beneficial to health whereas other types are capable of raising cholesterol levels and causing knock-on health problems. Fats can be categorized into two main types – saturated fat and unsaturated fat.

Saturated fat is believed to be implicated in the development of heart disease. It comes mainly from animal sources and is generally solid at room temperature. Although margarine was, for many years, believed to be a healthier choice than butter, nutritionists have now revised their opinion, for some of the fats in the margarine hydrogenation process are changed into trans-fatty acids, which the body metabolizes as if they were saturated fatty acids – the same as butter. Butter is a valuable source of oils and vitamin A, but should be used sparingly. Margarine, on the other hand, is an artificial product that contains many additives.

Unsaturated fat, also called polyunsaturated or monounsaturated fat, has a protective effect on the heart and other organs. Omega-3 and omega-6 oils occur naturally in oily fish, nuts and seeds. Unsaturated fat is usually liquid at room temperature. It is recommended, then, that women with PCOS should eat oily fish at least three times a week and cold-pressed oil (olive, rapeseed, safflower and sunflower oil) daily, for dressings and in cooking.

Olive oil is best suited to cooking, however, since it suffers less damage from heat than other oils.

Frying

The process of frying changes the molecular structure of foods, rendering them potentially damaging to the body. If you must fry something, it is best to use a small amount of extra-virgin olive oil and to cook at a low temperature. A healthier alternative is to sauté in a little water or tomato juice, or to grill, bake or steam. Stir-frying is good – but cook the food in a little water, drizzling on olive oil afterwards.

It is important to remember never to re-heat used oils, for this, too, can be harmful to the body. Store your oils in a sealed container in a cool, dark place to prevent rancidity.

Eggs

You are no doubt aware that eggs are high in cholesterol, which is a type of fat. However, they also contain lecithin, which is a superb biological detergent capable of breaking down fats so they can be utilized by the body – very useful for women with PCOS. Lecithin also prevents the accumulation of too many acid or alkaline substances in the blood and encourages the transportation of nutrients through the cell walls. Eggs should be soft-boiled or poached, since a hard yolk binds the lecithin, rendering it useless as a fat-detergent.

Although it is recommended that you eat two or three eggs a week, those following this diet on a vegetarian basis should eat up to five eggs a week to obtain the necessary protein.

A wholefood diet

Wholefoods are simply those which have had nothing taken away (nutrients or fibre) and that have had nothing added (colourings, flavourings or preservatives). In short, they are foods in their most natural form. Wholefoods that are organically produced, without the use of potentially dangerous chemical fertilizers, pesticides and herbicides, are even better for us.

The fibre in grains, fruit and vegetables is particularly beneficial in PCOS. Fibre reduces oestrogen levels by protecting the oestrogens secreted in the bile, effectively preventing them from being reabsorbed into the blood. Low-fat vegetarian foods are excellent since they help to speed up bowel transit time and so eliminate old oestrogens in the bowel.

A rough outline of the foods recommended follows.

Fresh fruit and vegetables

As well as helping to eliminate old oestrogens in the bowel, the high levels of fibre in fruit and vegetables also help to regulate insulin levels, as shown in several recent studies. Try to eat locally grown, organic foods that are in season. They have the highest nutrient content and the greatest enzyme activity. Enzymes are to our body what spark plugs are to the car engine. Without its 'sparks', the body doesn't work properly. Organically grown fruit and vegetables may not look so perfect as those that are processed, but they *are* superior – processed foods are devitalized of their 'sparks'.

Try to eat as fresh and as raw as possible – make a variety of salads and try to eat one every day. When you do cook vegetables, cook them in the minimum of unsalted (or lightly salted) water for the minimum of time. Lightly steaming or stir-frying are healthy alternatives. Scrub vegetables rather than peel them.

Legumes (peas and beans)

Although they contain high amounts of protein, legumes cost very little. The soya bean is a complete protein, and can be purchased as soya milk, tofu, tempeh and miso. Tofu, for example, is very versatile and can be used in both savoury and sweet dishes.

Because the soybean also contains phytoestrogens – that is, plant hormones that help to reduce high oestrogen levels (see below) – it is highly recommended for people with PCOS. Butter beans, mung beans, chick peas, haricot beans, lentils, garden peas, kidney beans and split peas are also rich sources of phytoestrogens and should be consumed as often as possible.

Seeds

Not only for the birds! Sunflower, sesame, hemp and pumpkin seeds contain a wonderful combination of nutrients, all of which are necessary to start a new plant and are also very important for normalizing the body's systems. They can be eaten as they are as a snack or sprinkled over salads and cereals, or they can be used in baking. For more flavour they can be lightly roasted and coated with organic soy sauce. Cracked linseed is also highly nutritious and it is useful for treating constipation. It can be used in baking and sprinkled over breakfast cereals and porridge oats. Flax, pumpkin and sesame seeds are particularly useful since they contain phytoestrogens.

Nuts

Nuts, too, should be an intrinsic part of your diet. All nuts contain vital nutrients, but almonds, cashew nuts, Brazil nuts and pecan nuts perhaps offer the greatest array. Eat a wide assortment as snacks, with cereals and in baking. Walnuts are excellent since they are high in phytoestrogens.

Grains

Wheat is our staple grain in the West, refined wheat flour being the product with which most of our cakes, pastries, biscuits and bread are made. However, refined wheat flour is not actually good for us – 'refined' meaning that the husks and germ have been removed and the remaining powder bleached. As a result, most of the nutritional value is removed, including the vitamins, minerals, protein and fibre. Only carbohydrates, calories and a little protein remain.

Fortified flours, as the name implies, have had some of their nutrients replaced. However, vitamin B6, vitamin E and folacin are not put back. Also, of the nine minerals initially removed, only three – iron, calcium and phosphorus – are returned, but in forms that are not easily absorbed by the body. All in all, refined flours have little nutritional value.

Healthy flours include wholewheat flour, spelt flour, quinoa flour, oat flour, maize flour, brown rice flour, rye flour, barley flour and potato flour, all of which are high in nutrients. Buckwheat, although not actually a grain, also makes a delicious alternative, and as with millet and rice, it is free of gluten, a common allergen. Because wheatgerm is high in the B vitamins that are so important to women with PCOS, it is highly recommended. Granary bread, to which crushed wheat and rye grains have been added, makes a pleasant alternative. Remember that organically produced flours are best.

A word of warning, however. Please ensure that your 'wholemeal' loaf of bread really *is* wholemeal and not made of dyed white flour or a mixture of flours. The word 'brown' in the description of a bread tells you nothing. Bread mixes that are nutritious and easy to prepare can be purchased in health-food shops.

You should aim to consume a variety of grains. Oats are highly recommended in PCOS as they help to stabilize blood sugar levels.

Phytoestrogens

A phytoestrogen is a naturally occurring plant nutrient – 'phyto' meaning plant – that exerts an oestrogen-like effect on the body. Studies have shown that the chemical structure of phytoestrogens is very close to human oestrogen and, while not as powerful as human oestrogen, they can play an important role in the healthy functioning of the human body. For example, if the body's oestrogen levels are low, as during the menopause, phytoestrogens will add to the body's oestrogen store. Alternatively, where oestrogen levels are high, as is often the case in PCOS, plant hormones can actually lower the body's oestrogen levels. They do this by competing with oestrogen for the 'binding sites' where oestrogen usually exerts its effect.

Scientists have discovered hundreds of edible phytoestrogens. They include soya beans, whole grain cereals, fennel, parsley, celery and flaxseed oil, as well as many nuts, seeds and herbs. The herbs known to be particularly useful for women with PCOS are black cohosh, red clover, dong quai, licorice, Korean ginseng and wild American ginseng.

Studies have shown that a phytoestrogen-rich diet can protect against endometrial cancer and can lower cholesterol levels. It is important to seek professional advice before taking any herbs during pregnancy.

A sample menu

To give you an idea of the type of foods recommended for women with PCOS, we have devised a 7-day sample menu. If this is very different to your current diet, please don't be daunted. This is an ideal, something that you might want to aim for over a period of time.

The drinks for this 'week' are not included in the plan, but they should include plenty of water, herbal teas and fresh fruit and vegetable juices. All fruit and vegetables should be organic, all bread wholemeal, and any pre-packaged foods should not contain additives.

Note that the cup you should use for the measures given below is a small teacup or American cup measure rather than a mug.

Day 1
Breakfast: Grapefruit with a little muscovado sugar and two slices of wholemeal toast
Snack: $\frac{1}{3}$ cup mixed sunflower seeds and almonds
Lunch: A salad of your choice, with low-fat mayonnaise but no cheese; an apple
Snack: $\frac{1}{3}$ cup dried apricots
Dinner: Irish stew with lean beef and plenty of vegetables
Snack: Two oatcakes (available from health-food shops)

Day 2
Breakfast: Porridge with cracked linseed, raw honey and rice milk
Snack: Banana
Lunch: Two soft-poached eggs on two slices of wholemeal toast
Snack: $\frac{1}{3}$ cup pecan nuts
Dinner: Grilled chicken breast with potatoes, carrots and green beans
Snack: An apple

Day 3
Breakfast: Grilled sardines on two slices of wholemeal toast
Snack: Carob bar (available from health-food shops)
Lunch: Bean and vegetable soup with two wholemeal rolls; a pear
Snack: $\frac{1}{3}$ cup mixed dried fruit and nuts
Dinner: Home-made chicken curry with brown rice
Snack: Two slices of wholemeal toast

Day 4
Breakfast: Large wedge of canteloupe melon
Snack: Two oatcakes
Lunch: Tuna salad; a banana
Snack: $\frac{1}{3}$ cup dried apricots
Dinner: Falafel (similar to a veggie-burger and available from health-food shops) with beans and home-made oven chips; an orange
Snack: $\frac{1}{3}$ cup mixed nuts

Day 5

Breakfast:	Porridge with cracked linseed, rice milk and a little muscovado sugar
Snack:	$\frac{1}{3}$ cup pecan nuts
Lunch:	Two grilled kippers with two slices of wholemeal bread
Snack:	Two kiwi fruit
Dinner:	Mixed vegetable casserole
Snack:	Two slices of wholemeal toast with raw honey

Day 6

Breakfast:	Fresh fruit salad
Snack:	Two crispbread biscuits with cottage cheese
Lunch:	Scotch broth; an apple
Snack:	$\frac{1}{3}$ cup mixed nuts
Dinner:	Tuna salad with two wholemeal rolls
Snack:	An orange

Day 7

Breakfast:	Two slices of wholemeal toast with raw honey
Snack:	Two rice cakes (available from health-food shops)
Lunch:	Mixed salad; baked apples
Snack:	A pear
Dinner:	Baked wild salmon with potatoes, broccoli and carrots
Snack:	Two oat cakes

Making changes

Changing the habits of a lifetime takes a lot of effort and determination. Eating is a pleasurable activity, we are used to choosing the foods that satisfy our taste buds (often made more tasty by the addition of chemical flavourings, fat, sugar, salt and so on) and we may be loath to make drastic changes. For these reasons, it is recommended that you alter your eating habits *gradually*, allowing yourself time to adjust to the new textures, appearances and flavours of different foods. With perseverance, your tastes *will* change – and as your PCOS symptoms decline, your interest in the new diet will probably increase!

If you wish to start eating the new foods straight away, we must add a word of warning, however. Nutritious, cleanly grown foods may trigger the body into instant detoxification, causing headaches, lethargy and even diarrhoea, lasting between 1 day and 2 weeks. You can avoid this shock to your system by a gradual changeover to healthier foods.

When starting to introduce the new diet, remember that it is important to eat a wide variety of foods. To eat the same things repeatedly means missing out on many vital building blocks of life, for certain foods build and regenerate only certain parts of the body.

If there are foods in the sample diet you just know you wouldn't eat on a regular basis, cut them out of your mind. A long-term diet will only work if it is practical, sustainable and compatible with your lifestyle. If you feel it would be too difficult to change over to healthy eating on your own, you may want to ask your doctor for a referral to a dietician for additional help. Alternatively, there are many excellent nutritionists who can offer skilled guidance, for a fee.

Retraining your palate

In comparison with the average Western diet, which has, by the addition of chemical flavourings, saturated fat, sugar and salt, evolved largely to please the taste buds, a healthy diet is based on foods in their more natural form. It is advisable, therefore, that you *slowly* retrain your palate to accept different tastes. For this reason, it is recommended that you cut back gradually on the amounts of sugar, salt and saturated fat that you consume. It takes only a month of eating a food regularly for it to become a habit.

Keeping a diary

Keeping a food-intake diary is an excellent way to monitor your progress. I suggest that you buy a notebook and devote a page to each day, listing all the foods you eat, including snacks and drinks.

Setting goals

It is a good idea to set small, achievable goals on the very first page of your diary – that way you should get quicker results. For example, you may wish to make a goal of eating two types of (organic) vegetables each day. Without the diary, you may assume you have done badly – but on reading your entries you may see that you have actually eaten two types of vegetables two or three times a week. That's a good starting point. Now you can focus on slowly increasing that amount.

Try not to make too many changes in too short a time. This is not a 'fad' diet you are trying, this is, we hope, a permanent lifestyle change, a step towards both weight loss and better health. Perhaps after setting a goal of eating more vegetables, you could set another to eat more fruit – again trying to buy organic fruit. After that, you could perhaps try to cut down on tea and coffee, instead drinking fruit juice, water and herbal teas. Cutting down on foods with additives could perhaps come next – with the eventual aim of eliminating them entirely.

Try not to count calories, though. You should soon feel the benefit in the fit of your clothes. Maybe you had better start saving for a whole new wardrobe of clothes for when you drop a dress size or two! Even if you are not overweight, an improved diet should have a positive impact on your PCOS.

Dietary supplements for women with PCOS

It is thought that anyone with a health problem is naturally deficient in certain vitamins and minerals. For that reason, women with PCOS may wish to take supplements. These generally come in tablet or capsule form, and can be purchased at health-food shops and specialist suppliers. They should be taken before meals to ensure maximum absorption. Look for supplements without added colourings, flavourings, preservatives, hydrogenated fats, gelatin and sugar – and check the strength with that of different brands. Sadly, some supplements contain only minute amounts of the active ingredients. A good company will have a qualified nutritionist available to answer telephone queries and will train retailers to know about their products. Of course, they may still be biased towards their own products.

Supplements for women with PCOS include the following.

- Chromium: studies have shown that chromium supplementation can improve glucose tolerance and the efficiency of insulin. Women with PCOS may wish to take up to 0.2 mg daily.

- B vitamins: these are known to aid the calming process and help the detoxification of the hormones for secretion from the body. Women with PCOS may wish to take up to 25 mg daily.
- A good anti-oxidant multivitamin–mineral combination. Anti-oxidants clean up the harmful 'free radicals' that come from sources such as industrial pollutants, ultraviolet light leaking in through the ozone layer, car exhaust fumes and smoking. They help the body at the important cellular level. Follow the dosage instructions on the label.
- Zinc, another anti-oxidant, aids in the maintenance of the reproductive organs. It also helps to correct insulin levels. Women with PCOS may wish to take up to 30 mg daily.
- Evening primrose oil: this essential fatty acid contains gamma-linolenic acid, which aids hormone balance. Women with PCOS may wish to take 500–1000 mg daily.

Water

Because water is required for most of the reactions in our bodies, a steady intake is essential (at least eight glasses a day). However, whether tap water is fit for human consumption is a matter for debate. Aluminium sulphate is added as a coagulant to ground water, then chemical polyelectrolites are put in to further settle the coagulated waste. Although this water is then passed through sand filters to remove the settled particles, many of the chemicals remain. This water is then combined with reservoir water, to which fluoride and chlorine are added. By the time it reaches our taps, it is loaded with inappropriate mineral salts and added chemicals. Other pollutants have often seeped in to contaminate it further.

As tap water may be of some detriment to people with PCOS, you may wish to use purified (filtered) water. This has the effect of detoxifying the harmful toxins in the environment and those ingested from processed foods. Water filters on the market vary from simple carbon filters to carbon filters with silver mesh components that even destroy bacteria. There are also reverse osmosis filters, which produce very clean water while still retaining some of the precious trace minerals. It must be said, however, that their individual effectiveness at removing pollutants is in proportion to their cost. Don't let this put you off, though – an inexpensive carbon filter is far better than no filter at all.

Oestrogens in the environment

Some of the chemicals in our environment are capable of altering hormone levels – they are known collectively as endocrine-disrupting chemicals. The result can be seen in some of the fish in our rivers, for their development has been greatly affected. It has been known for some years that a wide variety of chemicals are capable of disrupting the reproductive system by mimicking natural oestrogen, and in fish the effect can be seen in the development of female sexual organs in the male.

It must be assumed that these oestrogen mimics are having effects on humans too. This is seemingly evident in the dramatic drop in the male sperm count over the past 50 years. Half way through the last century the average sperm count was considered to be more than 60 million sperm per millilitre, whereas now the normal count is defined as above 20 million sperm per millilitre. As the incidence of menstrual disturbance, endometriosis, fibroids, infertility and breast cancer has almost tripled in the past 50 years, it can be assumed that endocrine-disrupting chemicals in the environment are at least partly to blame.

As processed foods contain endocrine-disrupting chemicals, it would be advisable to eat organic foods and cut down on your exposure to chemicals at home and in the workplace. Many personal care products contain endocrine-disrupting chemicals; however, natural products can now be obtained from high-street chemists and specialist manufacturers.

Exercise

As up to 50 per cent of the PCOS population are thought to be clinically obese, exercise is just as important as diet. Building up muscle mass and decreasing body fat can have a positive effect on many bodily functions. For instance, a lower body weight and reduced body fat percentage will raise levels of SHBG, which are generally low in women with PCOS. Higher levels of SHBG are advantageous as they reduce testosterone action. This, in turn, can decrease symptoms of hirsutism, acne and hair loss. Aerobic and weight-bearing exercise have the effect of reducing insulin resistance. Fat and muscle cells react more kindly to insulin in the blood, as a result of which the body needs to pump out less insulin to achieve the same response.

Warm-ups

It is important to warm up and mobilize the muscles and joints before embarking on aerobic and weight-bearing exercise. This will prepare the cardiovascular system for work by gradually increasing the body temperature and the blood flow to the working areas. Warm-ups also help to prevent muscular soreness and injury.

Stand with your feet about 40 cm (15 inches) apart, keep your body relaxed, your back straight, your bottom tucked in and your stomach flattened as you perform your routine. All exercises should be smooth and continuous.

- Shoulders: letting your arms hang loose, slowly circle your shoulders in a backwards motion. Repeat the exercise ten times. Now slowly circle your shoulders forwards and repeat ten times.
- Neck: slowly turn your head to the left then hold to a count of two. Return to the centre and repeat the exercise ten times. Now turn your head to the right then hold to a count of two before returning to the centre. Repeat ten times. Tucking in your chin, tilt your head down and hold to a count of two before returning to the centre. Repeat ten times. Finally, tilt your head upwards and hold to a count of two before returning to the centre. Repeat ten times.
- Spine (first set of warm-ups): placing your hands on your hips to help support your lower back, slowly tilt your upper body to the left and hold to a count of two. Return to the centre, and repeat between two and ten times. Now tilt to the right and return to the centre. Repeat between two and ten times (see Figure 3, opposite).
- Spine (second set of warm-ups): keeping your lower back static, swing your arms and upper body to the left as far as they will comfortably go, then return to the centre. Repeat ten times. Now swing your arms and upper body to the right and return to the centre. Repeat ten times.
- Hips and knees: with your body upright, move your hips by lifting your left knee upwards, as far as is comfortable. Hold to a count of two, then lower. Now raise your right knee and hold to a count of two. Repeat ten times (see Figure 4, opposite).
- Ankles: with your supporting leg slightly bent, place your left toes on the floor in front of you. Lift up your foot and then place your left heel on the floor. Repeat ten times. Now duplicate the exercise with the right foot (see Figure 5, p. 56).

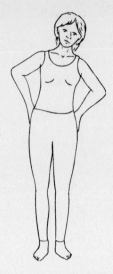

Figure 3 Warm-up exercise for the spine

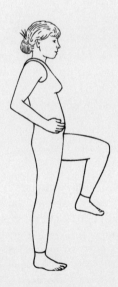

Figure 4 Warm-up exercise for the hips and knees

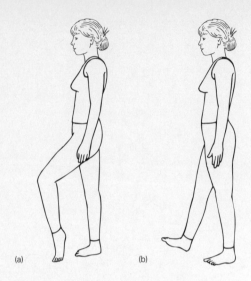

(a)   (b)

Figure 5 Warm-up exercises for the ankles

Pulse-raising activities

Pulse-raising activities, another part of your warm-up routine, should build up gradually. Their purpose is to warm your muscles further in preparation for stretching. Marching on the spot for 2–4 minutes, starting slowly, then speeding up a little more, is ideal.

Stretching exercises

Stretches prepare the muscles for the more challenging movements that will follow.

- Calf (first set of stretching exercises): stand with your arms outstretched and your palms against the wall. Keeping your left foot on the floor, bend your left knee. Press the heel of your right foot into the floor until you feel a gentle stretch in your leg muscles. Now change legs, alternating between the left and right leg. Repeat ten times (see Figure 6, opposite).
- Calf (second set of stretching exercises): standing with your feet slightly apart, raise both heels off the floor so that you are on your

56

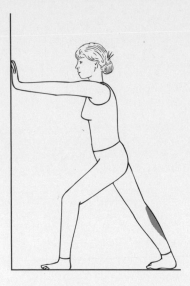

Figure 6 Stretching exercise for the calf

toes. Repeat ten times. As your calf muscles strengthen you should be able to stay on your toes for longer periods of time.

- Front of thigh: using a chair or the wall for support, stand with your left leg in front of your right, both knees bent, your right heel off the floor. Tuck in your bottom, and move your hip forwards until you feel a gentle stretch in the front of your right thigh. Now change legs. Repeat ten times (see Figure 7, overleaf).
- Back of thigh: stand with your legs slightly bent and your left leg about 20 cm (8 inches) in front of your right leg. Keeping your back straight, place both hands on your hips and lean forward a little. Now straighten your left leg, tilting your bottom upwards until you feel a gentle stretch in the back of your left thigh. Now change legs. Repeat ten times (see Figure 8, overleaf).
- Groin: spreading your legs slightly, your hips facing forward and your back straight, bend your left leg and move your right leg slowly sideways, keeping it straight, until you feel a gentle stretch in your groin. Gently move to the right, bending your right leg as you straighten the left (see Figure 9, p. 59).

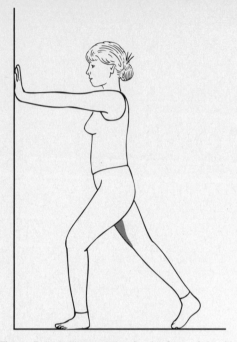

Figure 7 Stretching exercise for the front of the thigh

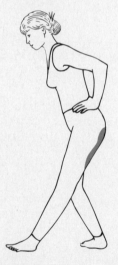

Figure 8 Stretching exercise for the back of the thigh

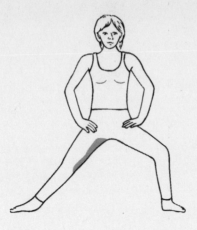

Figure 9 Stretching exercise for the groin

- Chest: keeping your back straight, your knees slightly bent and your pelvis tucked under, place your arms as far behind your lower back as you can. Now move your shoulders and elbows back until you feel a gentle stretch in your chest (see Figure 10, overleaf).

Aerobic exercise

Aerobic exercise – an activity that makes you slightly out of breath – should come next. This type of exercise is beneficial to women with PCOS since it improves cardiovascular function and helps to protect against high blood pressure (hypertension), heart disease and stroke. Regular aerobic activity carries the added bonus of releasing feel-good endorphins into your bloodstream, hence lifting your mood. It also aids overall fitness and the reduction of weight. Try to choose an activity that you will enjoy and want to continue.

Note that you should check with your doctor before embarking on regular aerobic activity.

- Walking: this most convenient, low-impact aerobic activity aids mobility, strength and stamina, and helps to protect against osteoporosis. You may find it easier to use a treadmill, reading a book or magazine at the same time or listening to a CD player, the

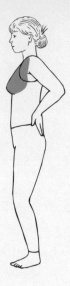

Figure 10 Stretching exercise for the chest

radio, or to story tapes. Try to walk for 20 or 30 minutes. A treadmill should never wholly replace outdoor walking.

- Stepping: start with a fairly small step (for example, a wide, hefty book, such as a catalogue or a telephone directory), or, if you wish, use a step machine or the bottom step of your staircase. Place first your left foot, then your right foot on to the book or step. Now step backwards, first with your left foot, then with your right foot. Repeat for 2–10 minutes, then change feet, placing first your right foot on to the step, then your left.

- Trampoline jogging: jogging on a small, circular trampoline can provide a good aerobic workout. If you can manage to get into a rhythm, the trampoline will do much of the work for you. Try to jog in this way for 20 or 30 minutes. Small, inexpensive trampolines are available from most exercise equipment outlets.

- Aqua aerobics: many people find aqua aerobics, sometimes called 'aqua-cizes', both easy and enjoyable. Because the water supports your body as you exercise, it removes the shock factor, conditioning your muscles with the very minimum of discomfort. The pressure of the water also causes the chest to expand, encouraging deeper breathing and increased intake of oxygen.

60

Rather than exercising alone in the swimming baths, most people prefer to join an aqua aerobics class. Most public swimming baths run aqua aerobic sessions, some of which are graded according to ability. As with all exercises, aqua aerobics are only truly beneficial when performed on a regular basis. If you live a long way from the swimming baths, you will probably find yourself attending less and less, then feel angry with yourself for eventually giving up. To minimize feelings of failure, be wary of undertaking activities that may be difficult to keep up.

- Swimming: if you enjoy swimming, try to go to the baths once or twice a week and gradually build up the number of lengths you swim. Swimming exercises every muscle in the body in a way that causes them very little stress. However, as with aqua aerobics or visiting a gym, you need to feel sure in yourself, before you start, that you will continue this type of exercise in the long term.
- Cycling: whether you use a stationary or an ordinary bicycle, this form of activity provides an efficient cardiovascular work-out. It is best to start by pedalling slowly and gradually building up momentum – and at first limit your sessions to 2 or 3 minutes, building up to 20 or 30 minutes, if possible.

Strength and endurance exercises

Strength and endurance exercises develop the muscles and help to raise levels of SHBG. As a result, the production of testosterone should gradually decline. If you feel that you have already done enough at this point, however, run through the warm-ups again as a way of cooling down, then congratulate yourself for doing something positive to help yourself. Perhaps when you feel fitter you can incorporate this section into your routine.

- Thighs (first set of strength and endurance exercises): lean back against the wall with your feet 30 cm (12 inches) away from the base of the wall. With your posture aligned, slowly squat down, keeping your heels on the ground. Now slowly straighten your legs again. Repeat between two and ten times.
- Thighs (second set of strength and endurance exercises): holding on to a sturdy chair and keeping your back 'tall', bend and then slowly straighten both legs, keeping your heels on the floor. Repeat the exercise between two and ten times (see Figure 11).

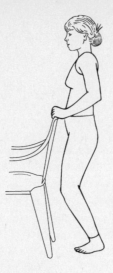

Figure 11 Exercise to strengthen the thigh

- Upper back: lie face down on the floor and, keeping your legs straight, gently raise your head and shoulders. Hold to a count of two, then lower them. Repeat between two and ten times (see Figure 12).

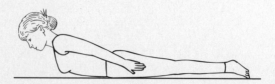

Figure 12 Exercise to strengthen the upper back

- Lower back: lie on your back and lift your right leg, pulling it towards your chest until you feel a gentle pull in your bottom and lower back. Repeat with the left leg. Now pull both legs up together. Repeat each exercise between two and ten times (see Figure 13, opposite).

- Abdomen: lie on your back with your knees bent and your feet flat on the floor. Now raise your head and shoulders, reaching with your arms towards your knees. Remember to keep the middle of your back on the floor (see Figure 14).

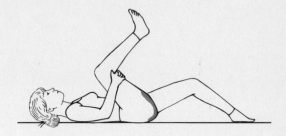

Figure 13 Exercise to strengthen the lower back

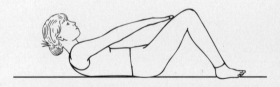

Figure 14 Exercise to strengthen the abdominal muscles

- Push-ups: stand with your hands flat against a wall, your body straight. Carefully lower your body towards the wall, then slowly push away. Repeat two to ten times (see Figure 15, overleaf).

Using weights

Exercising with weights can form part of your strength and endurance routine and will help you to lose any excess weight. You could use either a bag of sugar, a tin of baked beans, or the Velcro-fastening weights that fit around the wrists and ankles. It shouldn't be necessary to use anything heavier.

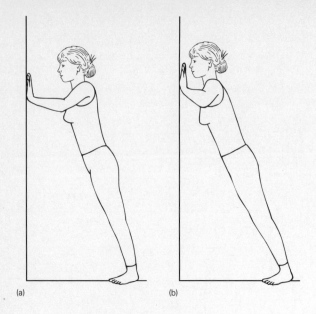

Figure 15 Push-ups against the wall

Fasten the weights around your wrists or hold firmly in each hand, then stand with your feet slightly apart. Now try the following exercises.

- Making sure that only your upper body moves, turn to the left, swinging both arms as you move. Repeat two or ten times. Now perform the same exercise and number of repetitions, swinging your body and arms to the right. Ensure the movements are slow and fluid. Build up the repetitions in line with your level of fitness.
- Keeping your left elbow close to your waist, slowly raise your left forearm so it almost touches your shoulder. Lower the arm until it is at right angles with your upper arm, then slowly raise it again. Ensure your movements are slow and continuous. Repeat between two and ten times.

64

- Bend your left arm so that your elbow is down and your forearm upright (in other words, so that your wrist is at your shoulder), then raise your arm upward until your elbow is straight. Bring it back down to the original position. Repeat once more, then do the same with your right arm. Repeat between two and ten times.

Cooling down

Finish your routine by cooling down, using the warm-up exercises given above.

Exercise routine

Ideally, you should carry out your routine three or four times a week. Try to exercise before eating breakfast, if possible. The low levels of insulin in your body at that time allow access to body fat for conversion to energy. To boost your fitness levels further – especially if you are not able to perform a regular aerobic regime – try walking to work, walking to the shops, getting off the bus a stop or two earlier and taking the stairs instead of the lift. Remember, most of all, that every little helps.

Managing stubborn symptoms

It can be frustrating to feel that you are doing your best to help yourself – taking the prescribed medications and following a healthy diet and exercise regime – only for the visible effects of PCOS stubbornly to remain. Unfortunately, it can take up to 18 months for problems like hirsutism, hair loss and acne to respond to medication, but in the mean time there are things that you can do to help yourself.

This section should also be of benefit to those who prefer not to use drug therapy to treat their PCOS.

Removing unwanted hair

There are several treatments available for removing unwanted hair. The following may help you to choose the method most suitable to you.

Electrolysis treatment

Electrolysis involves attending a local beauty salon or specialist clinic where a trained therapist inserts an ultra-thin probe into the hair follicle alongside the hair. A small amount of heat is delivered to the probe by a device known as an epilator. The cells that nourish the hair root are destroyed permanently, making regrowth weaker with time. Electrolysis is not considered a painful procedure. However, people have different levels of sensitivity and something that is comfortable for one person can cause discomfort to another. As tissue is being treated, a sensation of sorts is to be expected. Treatment may leave some redness which can last for a few hours.

Some women are referred by their doctor, endocrinologist or gynaecologist; others rely on the recommendation of a friend or simply look through the local telephone directory. To feel assured you are getting the best treatment, ask your electrologist whether he or she is licensed – licensing is required by law.

Depilatory creams

Application of chemical hair-removing cream causes hair that is visible to dissolve. Be sure to try out the cream on a hidden area of skin before using on the face since it can cause redness and soreness. It may even break the skin and should not be used where acne is present or where the skin is particularly sensitive. If there is persistent acne in the area requiring treatment, electrolysis is perhaps a better option. Depilatory creams remove only the surface hair, making regular application essential – and unfortunately, regrowth is inevitable because the hair root remains intact. The instructions on the label must be carefully followed.

Waxing

Waxing involves hot wax being spread by spatula over the skin. A cloth strip is pressed on to the wax and then pulled off with a quick movement that takes away the wax, hair and dead skin. Yes, this certainly stings! The skin is generally left smooth, but some people suffer redness and bumps, which disappear after a few hours. Because the hair is pulled out by the root, regrowth takes 3–8 weeks to become visible. Never apply wax to the nipples when removing hair from the breast area. Hair should be 3 mm ($\frac{1}{8}$ inch) long for this treatment to be successful. The skin should be pulled taut before the cloth strips are pulled away. Tough hair is easier to pull off. When waxing facial hair, use wax at a lower temperature and spread very thinly. If acne is a problem in the area requiring treatment, wait until the skin has healed before waxing to avoid further irritation. As with depilatory creams, electrolysis is perhaps the best option if acne is persistent. Moreover, if you are taking certain anti-acne medications, including tretinoin (also known as Retin-A or Renova), isotretinoin (also known as Accutane) and adapalene (also known as Differin), you are advised not to wax since these medications tend to weaken the skin, causing the skin to tear when the strips are removed. People with diabetes, poor circulation or varicose veins should also not use waxing to remove unwanted hair.

Waxing may be carried out either at a beauty salon or at home with the use of a home waxing kit purchased from a high street chemist.

Body sugaring is similar to waxing in that a sugar paste is applied to the skin. However, the paste needs only to be warm, not hot, and it sticks only to the hairs, making removal less painful. There is also less irritation with this type of treatment, which is offered by some salons.

Shaving

Perhaps the easiest option of all, shaving can be used virtually everywhere but on the face. Wash the area thoroughly with water as hot as you can bear before applying plenty of soap. Shave with a clean blade and try to resist using your partner's razor – it is likely to cause reddening and an unsightly rash. Rinse the area thoroughly afterwards. Battery-operated shavers may also be used. It is not advisable, however, to shave in sensitive areas, such as around the nipples. Because shavers and razors only remove hair at skin level, regrowth will probably be rapid.

Bleaching

Bleaching is a 'concealing' treatment that works well for women whose hair on the head is not too dark. Cream bleaches for facial and body hair are available from high-street chemists and take only a few minutes to work. Many of these preparations contain aloe vera and vitamin E to soothe the skin. Follow the instructions on the label carefully.

Laser and photothermolysis

In recent years there has been a great deal of progress in the use of laser and photothermolysis hair-removing techniques. They look promising and are much faster and more effective than shaving, waxing and chemical depilation. Repeated treatments are required for a near-permanent effect because only hair follicles in the growing phase are obliterated at each treatment. Hair growth occurs in three cycles, so 6–9 months of regular treatments are typical. Unfortunately, this is an expensive option and is really suitable only for fair-skinned women with dark hair.

Persistent hair loss

If your hair is thinning, there are now many cosmetic products on the market that can make it appear thicker. If your hair is particularly thin at the crown, choose either a swept-back style or put your hair up to cover the area. Hair that is receding at the front is more difficult to conceal, and hair volumizing products may be your best course of action. An improved diet, stress management, drug therapy or use of the herbal remedy Agnus castus (also known as Agnolyt) can bring back hair growth. Sometimes it is helpful to have hair extensions, although these can be costly and need to be replaced on a regular basis.

Persistent acne

If you have a problem with acne that is not responding to treatment, try the following suggestions.

- Drink plenty of water. In order to detoxify your system and help the spots to retreat, try to drink between six and eight glasses of pure water a day. Distilled water is the best option; however, it is not always readily available. Portable water purifiers, available from supermarkets and many high street shops, can be an inexpensive option. Drinking cool boiled water is another useful alternative.
- Eat a well-balanced diet that contains plenty of fruit, vegetables, oily fish, nuts, seeds and grains; this will also help to improve your complexion.
- Tea tree oil can be beneficial, since it contains over a hundred natural anti-fungal, anti-bacterial and anti-viral properties.

- Hemp oil can be useful as a skin cream, since it contains omega-6 fatty acids, which have been found to be effective in the treatment of acne.
- Sarsaparilla is not only useful for helping to redress the hormonal balance, it also is capable of reducing acne.
- Echinacea, a natural 'antibiotic', can help to improve acne, as can calendula (marigold cream) and goldenseal.

Persistent obesity

If you are having difficulties in losing weight, try to take note of the following suggestions.

- Motivate yourself to follow a balanced diet by telling yourself that not only will you lose weight, but your other PCOS symptoms are likely to improve too. If you hope to get pregnant, losing weight will increase your chances of conceiving.
- Eat plenty of the foods that you are allowed (see above). Remember that saturated fats and refined carbohydrates raise insulin levels and cause fat to be stored in the fat cells. Make sure you have plenty of healthy snacks. Allow yourself an occasional treat to make the diet easier to cope with.
- Take plenty of exercise. Try to follow an exercise regime for 3–4 days a week, starting with warm-ups and going on to small weights and an aerobic activity – something that makes you slightly out of breath (see above). If you really can't face an exercise regime, try to walk to and from work or to and from school or the shops as often as you can. You will feel pleased with yourself each time you do so. More importantly, it will help to firm your muscles and lose the fat.
- Take a close look at your wardrobe. If you are keeping 'thin' clothes as an incentive to lose weight, it is unlikely to work. These clothes are a constant reminder of the weight you've put on and are likely to make you feel guilty. Take along a friend who is not afraid to speak her mind when you next go shopping for clothes. Don't necessarily stick to items that feel comfortable; rather look for clothes that help you to feel feminine too. Baggy tops can make you appear larger than ever. Try on something that is not exactly clingy, but that skims your figure. You may be pleasantly surprised! Avoid horizontal stripes, choosing vertical instead. Women with larger breasts can look top-heavy in high-necked

tops. Try something with a lower neckline and you may be surprised at the effect. And why not show off those very feminine assets? There are plenty of women who would adore larger breasts.

- Stand proud. Improving your posture, standing tall and holding back your shoulders can alter other people's impression of you. If you give off an air of confidence, others are more likely to treat you with the respect you deserve. An upright posture also has the effect of making you appear slimmer.

6

Complementary Treatments

As well as improving your diet and environment and starting an exercise regime, there are many other things you can do to help yourself. This chapter discusses the treatments available in addition to orthodox medicine.

Remember to inform your doctor if you wish to embark on a particular complementary therapy.

Complementary medicine

Complementary medicine has been described as 'all the therapies not taught in medical school'. These therapies include acupuncture, aromatherapy, homoeopathy and reflexology. You may know these techniques as 'alternative therapies', but this term can be misleading. The word 'alternative' suggests they can be used in place of conventional medicine, when that is not the intention. As with treating other disorders, complementary therapies in PCOS should be used in conjunction with the treatment and advice of your own doctor. Perhaps one of the main benefits of complementary therapies is that the therapist is able to spend time with the patient and can therefore lend more support than can be provided by the over-stretched NHS hospital or GP clinics.

Complementary therapies are suitable for women with PCOS for the following reasons:

- because of their non-invasive qualities,
- they are largely free from side-effects,
- they can be used in addition to long-term medication, and
- most of the therapies are enjoyable – the 'patient' can often completely relax, especially with the touch and massage techniques.

People who use complementary therapies often report benefits, although that may be partly because they know they are doing something positive to help themselves. Different therapies seem to suit different people.

Acupuncture

An ancient form of oriental healing, acupuncture involves puncturing the skin with fine needles at specific points in the body. These points are located along energy channels (meridians) that are believed to correspond to specific internal organs. This energy is known as chi. Needles are inserted to increase, decrease or unblock the flow of chi energy so that the balance of yin and yang is restored.

Yin, the female force, is calm and passive; it also represents dark, cold, swelling and moisture. On the other hand, yang, the male force, is stimulating and aggressive, representing heat, light, contraction and dryness. It is thought that an imbalance in these forces is the cause of illness and disease. A person who feels the cold, suffers fluid retention and has fatigue would be considered to have an excess of yin. A person who suffers from headaches and irritation, however, would be deemed to have an excess of yang.

Emotional, physical or environmental factors are believed to disturb the chi energy balance, and these can also be treated. For example, acupuncture has been used to alleviate stress, digestive disorders, insomnia, asthma and allergy. In some cases, it is thought to be capable of kick-starting menstrual periods and helping to regulate the menstrual cycle in women with PCOS.

A qualified acupuncturist will use a set method to determine acupuncture points – it is thought there are as many as 2000 acupuncture points on the body. At a consultation, questions will be asked about your lifestyle, sleeping patterns, fears, phobias, and reactions to stress. You will also be asked about your particular health problems. Your pulses will be taken, then the acupuncture itself carried out. Women with PCOS can expect to have needles placed in points in the arms, legs and abdomen. The acupuncturist will normally work on the liver chi and spleen chi to treat abnormal bleeding. Some people experience a stinging sensation as the needle goes in, others report feeling barely any discomfort. The first consultation will normally last for an hour, and patients should notice improvements after four to six sessions. If no benefits are noted, it may be best to discontinue treatment. (For details of the British Acupuncture Council, see the Useful Addresses section on page 99.)

Aromatherapy

Aromatherapy is the utilization of our sense of smell in the treatment of certain health disorders. Aromatherapists work to normalize the hormonal imbalances in PCOS and to aid relaxation and the release of emotional stress. Concentrated aromatic oils – also known as essential oils – are extracted from plants and may be inhaled, rubbed directly into the skin or used in bathing.

Plant essences have been used for healing throughout the ages, smaller amounts being used for aromatherapy purposes than for herbal medicines. The highly concentrated aromatherapy oils are obtained either by steaming a particular plant extract until the oil glands burst, or by soaking the plant extract in hot oil so that the cells collapse and release their essence.

Techniques used in aromatherapy

There are three main techniques used in aromatherapy – inhalation, massage and bathing.

Effecting the quickest result, inhalation of essential oils has a direct influence on the olfactory (nasal) organs and the aromas are immediately received by the brain. Steam inhalation is perhaps the most popular technique. Mix a few drops of oil with a bowlful of boiling water, or use an oil burner whereby a tea-light candle heats a small container of water and a few drops of oil.

Essential oils intended for massage are normally pre-diluted. These oils should never be applied directly to the skin in an undiluted (pure) form. When using undiluted essential oils, mix three or four drops with a neutral carrier oil, such as olive oil or safflower oil. The oils penetrate the skin and are absorbed by the body, exerting a positive influence on a particular organ or set of tissues.

Tension and anxiety can also be reduced by using specific aromatherapy oils in the bath. A few drops of pure essential oil should be added directly to running tap water. It disperses and mixes more efficiently this way. No more than 20 drops of oil in total should be added to bathwater.

The oils thought to be particularly useful for women with PCOS are as listed below. Each oil can either be used in the bath or in a burner or else mixed with a carrier oil and massaged into the skin.

- Lavender is the most popular oil for use in the bath. It is a wonderful restorative and excellent for relieving tension headaches as well as stress.
- Ylang ylang has relaxing properties. It has a calming effect on the heart rate and can be used to relieve palpitations and raised blood pressure.
- Chamomile can be very soothing. It aids both sleep and digestion, and it has anti-inflammatory properties.
- Jasmine is a renowned aphrodisiac and can reawaken passion and ease sexual problems. It encourages the expression of pleasure and affection. It has a powerful aroma, so use it in small doses.
- Bergamot lifts the spirits and can aid depression, anxiety and insomnia. Its nature is to balance the body and instil composure. If using it as a massage oil, do not apply before exposure to the sun since this may cause irritation to sensitive skin.
- Cedar gives strength at times of crisis. It calms and soothes nervous tension and anxiety. Its nature is to remind us of our own inner strength. Avoid this oil during pregnancy.
- Rose oil is said to bring warmth to the soul. It helps to heal emotional wounds and restores the trust that makes it possible for us to love ourselves.
- Sandalwood oil acts as a gentle sedative that has an uplifting effect on the psyche.

As aromatherapy is a holistic treatment (where the practitioner looks at the person and their ills as a whole), questions on lifestyle, family circumstances and so on will be asked at a consultation. Depending on your answers, a suitable essential oil (or more than one oil) will be recommended. As well as being of benefit to your health, aromatherapy massages can be very relaxing.

If you would prefer not to consult with a qualified aromatherapist, your local health-food store may be able to provide you with further details of the essential oils that are appropriate to your needs. In addition, you may wish to borrow a good aromatherapy book from your nearest library.

Bach flower remedies

In the 1930s, the philosophy of a Harley Street doctor, Edward Bach (pronounced 'batch'), was that 'a healthy mind ensures a healthy body'. He was a man far ahead of his time, considering that it is only in recent years we have concluded that the mind and body are closely linked.

Dr Bach devised a method of treating the negative emotional state behind any disorder. First, he sectioned emotional states into seven major groups, then he categorized 38 negative states of mind under each group. Using his knowledge of homoeopathy, he went on to formulate a plant- or flower-based remedy to treat each.

Fear

For terror he formulated 'rock rose' remedy.
For fear of known things he formulated 'mimulus'.
For fear of mental collapse he formulated 'cherry plum'.
For fears and worries of unknown origin he formulated 'aspen'.
For fear or over-concern for others he formulated 'red chestnut'.

Loneliness

For impatience he formulated 'impatiens'.
For self-centredness/self-concern he formulated 'heather'.
For pride and aloofness he formulated 'water violet'.

Insufficient interest in present circumstances

For apathy he formulated 'wild rose'.
For lack of energy he formulated 'olive'.
For unwanted thoughts or mental arguments he formulated 'white chestnut'.
For lack of interest in the present he formulated 'clematis'.
For deep gloom with no known origin he formulated 'mustard'.
For failure to learn from past mistakes he formulated 'chestnut bud'.
For people living in the past he formulated 'honeysuckle'.

Despondency or despair

For extreme mental anguish he formulated 'sweet chestnut'.
For self-hatred or a sense of uncleanliness he formulated 'crab apple'.
For over-responsibility he formulated 'elm'.
For lack of confidence he formulated 'larch'.
For self-reproach or guilt he formulated 'pine'.
For after-effects of shock he formulated 'star of Bethlehem'.

For resentment he formulated 'willow'.

For those feeling exhausted but struggling on he formulated 'oak'.

Uncertainty

For hopelessness and despair he formulated 'gorse'.

For despondency he formulated 'gentian'.

For indecision he formulated 'scleranthus'.

For uncertainty as to the correct path in life he formulated 'wild oat'.

For the seeker of advice and confirmation from others he formulated 'cerato'.

For 'Monday morning' feeling he formulated 'hornbeam'.

Over-sensitivity to influences and ideas

For weak will and subserviency he formulated 'centaury'.

For mental torment behind a brave face he formulated 'agrimony'.

For hatred, envy or jealousy he formulated 'holly'.

For protection from change and outside influences he formulated 'walnut'.

Over-care for the welfare of others

For intolerance he formulated 'beech'.

For over-enthusiasm he formulated 'vervain'.

For self-repression/self-denial he formulated 'rock water'.

For the selfishly possessive he formulated 'chicory'.

For dominance and inflexibility he formulated 'vine'.

In addition, the famous 'rescue remedy' is appropriate to many everyday situations in which emotional upheaval occurs. It is made up from a combination of five Bach flower remedies (rock rose, clematis, cherry plum, impatiens and star of Bethlehem).

Place a few drops of your chosen remedy on your tongue, or dilute it in water.

Herbal remedies

Traditional Chinese herbal remedies have been used, to great effect, since antiquity – and they are still the most widely used medicines in the world. In fact, 30 per cent of modern conventional medicines are made from plant-derived substances. However, because conventional medicines frequently carry toxic side-effects, herbal medicines are preferred by many people. Indeed, they seem to rate among the most popular of complementary therapies for women with PCOS.

Although they are natural, herbal medicines should be used with caution because they are capable of interacting with prescribed medications. You should always inform your doctor of what you are taking. Indeed, many doctors believe herbal medicine should not be taken without the advice of a trained herbalist. Your chosen herbalist will check your pulse rate and the colour of your tongue for clues as to which bodily organs are energy-depleted. He or she will then write a prescription for very precise dosages according to your needs. Tablets made from compressed herbal extracts are often supplied, but sometimes patients are given a bag of carefully weighed and ground dried roots, flowers, bark and so on, together with full instructions.

Various herbs are considered useful for treating PCOS. Please note, though, that there have never been any adequately powered, prospective randomized scientific studies that have assessed their validity.

Agnolyt

Agnus castus (also known as Agnolyt) has a long history of use for female hormone regulation. Its apparent effectiveness comes about because it works on the pituitary gland, which stimulates the hormones involved in reproduction. The secret of the success of this preparation appears to be that a tincture is made from the fruit of Agnus castus rather than from other parts of the shrub, unlike most other herbal formulations. Taken over 6–8 months, Agnolyt appears to be capable of stimulating the pituitary gland sufficiently that it normalizes the menstrual cycle, increasing levels of progesterone and LH and balancing progesterone and oestrogen production. This can have the result of making pregnancy achievable.

Agnolyt is a member of the family of adaptogenic herbs, which means they are able to adapt to the particular needs of the body. It must be said, though, that taking too much of this herb can cause depression. Women with PCOS should start on 30 drops once a day in the morning and reduce the dosage to 25 or even 20 drops if they start to feel low. Agnolyt can be obtained from specialist supplement manufacturers. (Contact details can be found in the Useful Addresses section on page 99.)

Rhodiola rosea

Rhodiola rosea is a powerful Russian nutrient that also belongs to the family of adaptogenic herbs. For people who feel stressed, this herb can encourage the body to adapt. Research has shown that Rhodiola rosea can boost sexual function, help to raise energy levels, increase resistance to disease and aid the detoxification of hormones before they are eliminated from the body. It is also believed to have revitalizing properties and can help to stabilize mood swings.

Most health-food shops now stock this stress-busting adaptogen, as do specialist supplement manufacturers. (See the Useful Addresses section on page 99 for further details.)

Ashwagandha

Also an adaptogenic herb, ashwagandha – sometimes called Indian ginseng – is an important tonic, containing a broad range of important healing powers rare in the plant kingdom. Not only is it good for restoring energy in people who often feel tired, it has also been shown in research to help to ease insomnia and stress.

In one study of 101 subjects, the indications of ageing – such as greying hair and low calcium levels – were found to be significantly improved in those taking ashwaganda.[18] Seventy per cent of the subjects in this study also reported increased libido and sexual function.

Ashwagandha can be found in most health-food shops and is available from specialist supplement manufacturers.

Siberian ginseng

The many benefits of Siberian ginseng – the most well known of the adaptogenic herbs – are said to include increased physical endurance under stress, improved hormone activity and better sexual function. This very safe herb is available from most health-food shops and specialist supplement manufacturers.

Sarsaparilla

Sarsaparilla is useful for helping to redress a hormonal imbalance. It contains a steroid-like substance that acts in a similar way to progesterone in the body. It is believed to stimulate the reproductive organs and have a tonic-like effect on the sex organs. Sarsaparilla is also capable of reducing acne.

White peony

White peony is useful for women with PCOS since it can help to normalize androgen levels in the body. It is also thought to reduce irritability and stress.

Echinacea

One of the most widely researched of all the herbs, echinacea has broad antibiotic properties, much like penicillin, and as such can be useful for treating acne. Alcohol-free tinctures are now available in most health-food shops.

St John's wort

St John's wort is probably the most successful natural antidepressant. Studies have shown that it works by increasing the action of the chemical serotonin and by inhibiting depression-promoting enzymes. Similar effects are created by drugs such as fluoxetine (also known as Prozac) and phenelzine (also known as Nardil), which carry a high risk of side-effects. St John's wort, however, has the happy advantage of being virtually free of side-effects. (In some cases it can produce a stomach upset, but this should stop within a few days.)

One study has indicated that St John's wort encourages sleep, and another that it benefits the immune system. In Germany, this herb outsells Prozac by three to one, and is said to be just as effective for treating mild depression. Because of its anti-inflammatory and anti-viral properties, it can also be useful for treating acne. It helps fight viral infections too.

Because your skin may be more sensitive to the sun's rays when you are taking this herb, don't forget to use a good sun-blocker.

Other herbal remedies

German chamomile, lavender, lemon balm and vervain are also effective herbal remedies that can ease emotional stress.

Homoeopathy

The homoeopathic approach to medicine is holistic (in other words, the overall health of a person – physical, emotional and psychological – is assessed before treatment commences). The homoeopathic belief is that the whole make-up of a person determines the disorders to which he or she is prone and the symptoms that are likely to occur. After a thorough consultation, the homoeopath will offer a remedy compatible with the patient's symptoms as well as with their temperament and characteristics. Consequently, two people with the same disorder may be offered entirely different remedies.

Homoeopathic remedies are derived from plant, mineral and animal substances, which are soaked in alcohol to extract what are known as the 'live' ingredients. This initial solution is then diluted many times, being vigorously shaken to add energy at each dilution. Impurities are removed and the remaining solution is made up into tablets, ointments, powders or suppositories. Low-dilution remedies are used for severe symptoms, while high-dilution remedies are used for milder symptoms.

Nowadays, homoeopathic remedies can be formulated to aid virtually every disorder. However, although the remedies are safe and non-addictive, the patient's symptoms may briefly worsen. This is known as a 'healing crisis' and is usually short-lived. It is actually an excellent indication that the remedy is working well.

Unfortunately, it is a common misconception that you can just pop along to your local chemist, look up your particular complaint on the homoeopathic remedy chart, begin taking the remedy and see marvellous results. If only it were as simple as that! Homoeopathic training takes several years, and a lot of knowledge and experience is required before practitioners can decide the correct remedies for complaints other than the very superficial. And, as mentioned earlier, what works for one person is not liable to work for another.

Selecting an appropriate remedy is only part of the procedure, however. The homoeopath will also evaluate the patient's reaction to ascertain what, if any, further treatment is necessary. Some women with PCOS have reported that their menstrual cycle normalized within 6 to 9 months after they began taking prescribed homoeopathic remedies. However, this information comes from uncontrolled clinical trials and the benefits of homoeopathy on women with PCOS have never been properly studied.

Reflexology

Reflexology, an ancient oriental therapy, has only recently been adopted in the Western world. It operates on the proposition that the body is divided into different energy zones, all of which can be exploited in the prevention and treatment of any disorder.

Reflexologists have identified ten energy channels, beginning in the toes and extending to the fingers and the top of the head. Each channel relates to a particular bodily zone, and to the organs in that zone. For example, the big toe relates to the head (the brain, sinus area, neck, pituitary gland, eyes and ears). By applying pressure to the appropriate terminal in the form of a specialized massage, a practitioner can determine which energy pathways are blocked. Minute lumps – like crystalline deposits – detected beneath the skin are then broken up by steady pressure. The theory is that the deposits are absorbed into the body's waste disposal system and removed through sweat or urine, hence restoring the correct energy flow.

Experts in this type of manipulative therapy claim that all the organs of the body are reflected in the feet. They also believe that reflexology aids the removal of waste products and blockages within the energy channels, improving circulation and glandular function. Reflexology is certainly relaxing, and it aids the release of stress. It is said to be able to help to regulate the menstrual cycle too.

Many therapists prefer to take a full case history before starting treatment. Each session will take up to 45 minutes (the preliminary session may take longer), and you will be treated either sitting in a chair or lying down.

7

Emotional Support

It is unfortunate that the many physical aspects of PCOS carry with them emotional repercussions. This chapter offers advice and coping techniques to help you to overcome these problems.

Your appearance

Many of the symptoms of PCOS can focus your attention on your appearance. When acne persists beyond young adulthood or when the hair on your head starts to thin in your 20s or 30s, it is doubtless both embarrassing and frustrating, as is a darkening or thickening of facial or body hair and putting on weight. To discover on top of other symptoms that you may have difficulty conceiving or, if you have been trying for a baby, that you are classed as infertile can be heartbreaking. Unfortunately, it is a fact that the symptoms of PCOS can attack a woman's sense of femininity; they can strike a blow at the very heart of who and what she is.

It is no wonder, then, that women with PCOS can lose their confidence. Some even become depressed. All people have doubts about their appearance and areas of their bodies they don't really like, but in PCOS it can seem that nature is conspiring against you, for often there may be many problem areas in evidence. It is not easy to fight a negative self-image, though, especially when the low moods take hold – but you only have one go at life, and you owe it to yourself and the people who are close to you to make the very most of it.

To give you a kick-start in raising your spirits, perhaps you could embark on a course of one of the 'stress-busting' herbal remedies mentioned in Chapter 6 – preferably with the guidance of a trained herbalist. In addition, you could start a course of one of the other beneficial complementary therapies, the ultimate aim being to reduce your PCOS symptoms. Your improved mood and the feeling that you are helping yourself should, we hope, provide the boost you need to tackle the emotional effects of the disorder.

The following pointers should help you to feel less negative about your body image.

- Try to stop looking back on those 'rosy days' when your body may have been more to your liking. Looking back can only cause further emotional pain, and that's the last thing you need right now. Letting go of the past and trying to live in the present can give you the strength to tackle the problems that you can do something about, such as losing weight and embarking on a course of electrolysis treatments.
- Try to accept the things that you can't change. Fortunately, in PCOS diet, exercise, stress management and drug therapy can reduce or even eradicate the symptoms. However, there may be areas that are stubborn, such as thinning hair or acne. If you are doing everything you can to improve your health, try not to become frustrated when there is little or no change. Keep on trying, though – it can take many months for the benefits to be really seen. Talk to your doctor too – he or she may be able to offer more help.
- Cheer yourself up by changing your image. A new hairstyle and perhaps a new hair colour can work wonders where confidence is concerned, as can a few changes to your wardrobe. Treat yourself to a facial, an aromatherapy massage, some new make-up. Instead of trying to hide yourself away, make the most of yourself. A brighter outside can cheer you up on the inside.
- Share your worries. Confide in someone close about your concerns over your body image. You will probably find that this person, too, has concerns about herself that you had not even guessed at. If you feel you are deeply affected by the way you look, it may be best to seek the help of a qualified counsellor. Your doctor should be able to make a recommendation.
- Take regular exercise. Walking, cycling and swimming are just three examples of activities that raise levels of the feel-good endorphins – the natural hormones that give you a lift. Feeling that you have done something good for yourself will help to put you in a positive frame of mind.

Boosting confidence and self-esteem

A person who dislikes his or her appearance will automatically have low self-esteem. Whether the problem is one particular part of the body or several areas, the effect is the same. A woman with PCOS may start by trying to hide a particular part of herself – but at some point she will realize that she is not really succeeding, as a result of which she may stop making any effort with her appearance. This has a further detrimental effect. There are some useful techniques, however, that can be employed to counter the negative feelings.

Self-talk

The way we speak to ourselves has a great bearing on our self-esteem and stress levels. When we analyse our thoughts, we are often surprised at their negativity – but they must be examined before we can begin to change their destructive pattern. If we drop something, we might think, 'I'm really clumsy'. If we make an error adding up, we might think, 'I'm useless at maths'. The same goes if we dislike a particular aspect of our appearance – except in this instance we might think, 'I'm worthless because I'm fat,' or 'I'm not feminine – therefore I'm a freak'. In cases where a relationship is involved, a woman with PCOS might even tell herself she is unworthy of her partner's affections. Unfortunately, such negative self-talk serves only to affirm your deepest fears about yourself.

To boost your self-esteem, try to catch yourself every time you have a negative thought about yourself – and instead, counter the thought with one that is positive, for there is sure to be something about your appearance that you can feel happy about. Be completely honest, now. Look at yourself in a full-length mirror and really *see* the positive things. Then maybe you could tell yourself, 'I am shapely and have a nice firm bottom,' or 'I am voluptuous and have good legs,' or 'I have pretty eyes, good hair and a nice, cuddly figure'.

Smile for a while

'All things are cause either for laughter or weeping,' wrote the Roman philosopher, Seneca. It is true that comedy and tragedy are close bedfellows, for both are reflex actions rooted in the central nervous system and its related hormones.

How we respond to certain stimulus, however, depends on our outlook on life. Letting go of the past and our fears for the future is 'releasing'. It allows us to smile more. Laughing at ourselves in particular can be more therapeutic than a whole-body massage; it can be more releasing than sex or alcohol, and it invariably makes other people warm to us. When we laugh, our muscles relax, bleak thoughts lift, and 'feel-good' endorphins are released into our bloodstream. As a result, we feel uplifted and bright!

However, as we go about our daily routines, we often forget to smile and laugh. Try to make a point of watching funny films and TV comedies, spend time with someone who lifts your spirits, read books that make you smile, and make a determined effort to see the funny side of things. Force yourself to laugh out loud every day – preferably when you are home alone. The laughter will quickly become real and you will feel so much better for doing something that felt so silly at first!

List the positive things

When you feel low, take a pen and paper and write down all the good things in your life. They could be such things as a job you enjoy, a loyal best friend, some great nights out, that old lady who always smiles at the bus stop, the neighbour who often stops for a chat, your dog who gets so excited when you come home . . . See what I mean?

Now make a list of all the good things about yourself. Think hard now. There will be a lot more than you might have realized. You may be a good listener, a good cook, have a pleasant singing voice, a good fashion sense, a good sense of direction, a great sense of humour. Don't stop writing until you are sure you've not missed a thing. Now read each item again, quite slowly, and really absorb the pleasure that doing so brings.

Helping those close to you to understand

In attempting to help the people you care about to understand the challenges you face with PCOS, you should try to be as honest and open as possible. It's far from easy to speak about the defeminizing nature of the condition in particular, so think first about what you want to say. The following pointers should help you.

Communicating effectively

Before endeavouring to describe your feelings about your disorder, you first need to focus on how you do actually feel. It will probably be hard to admit to feeling guilty, frustrated, angry, resentful, useless and so on, even to yourself, but doing so will help you to come to terms with those feelings and ultimately to let them go. Sharing your feelings with others, meanwhile, is an important step towards halting the problems those feelings can cause.

In your interactions with others, it is important that you try to be wary of making assumptions about how they feel about you. For instance, speaking to someone in the following way is sure to make that person feel that he or she is being unfairly judged: 'I know you think I'm worrying over nothing and that makes me really upset', or 'I don't believe you could really love someone who's hairy and spotty, and that makes me feel so bad', or 'You could try to diet with me. Seeing you eat all that food makes me feel like not bothering.' Such comments are likely to be seen as accusations; they may even provoke a quarrel.

Speaking directly of your 'emotional problems' – but without implying that the other person is contributing to those problems – will help the other person to take your comments more seriously. It should encourage him or her to be more thoughtful and caring. However, there may be times when conflict arises, when someone upsets you by doing or saying something hurtful. In such instances, the following list of considerations could be taken into account before you make your reply.

- Ensure you have interpreted the other person's behaviour correctly. For example, you may view your mother's bringing you a basket of fruit and vegetables as a criticism of your diet – when in truth it is a goodwill gesture, just to show that she cares. You have a perfect right to interpret the words or actions of others in whatever way you wish, but that interpretation is not necessarily reality. In fact, it is amazing how wrong we often are in our perceptions of what others think and feel.
- Ensure you are specific in recalling another person's behaviour. For example, 'You never understand when I tell you I feel less feminine than I used to' is far more inflammatory than 'You didn't seem to understand yesterday when I said I don't feel as feminine as I used to.'
- Ensure that what you are about to say is what you really mean. For example, statements such as 'Everyone thinks you're insensitive' or 'We all think you've got an attitude problem' are, besides being inflammatory, incredibly unfair. We have no way of

knowing that 'everyone' is of the same opinion. The use of the depersonalized 'everyone', 'we' or 'us' – often said in the hope of deflecting the listener's anger – can cause far more hurt and anger than if the criticism was direct and personal.

It is easy to see how others can misunderstand or take offence when we fail to communicate effectively. Changing the habits of a lifetime is far from easy, however. It means analysing our thoughts before rearranging them into speech. We are rewarded for our efforts, though, when those close to us start to really listen, when they cease to be annoyed as we carefully explain something they hadn't fully understood.

Dealing with unfair comments

Sarcastic and derisory remarks from others can chip away at your confidence. They should not, therefore, pass unchallenged. Standing up for yourself is not always easy, but doing so can have a releasing effect – unlike when you fake indifference, or clam up and walk away. In such instances, you may end up feeling hurt, offended and very resentful. Your most intense feeling, however, will probably be that of anger – at the other person, and at yourself, for allowing yourself to be hurt.

For example, if your partner were to say, 'You've put on so much weight ... you're not the woman I married', you could calmly answer, 'That's a hurtful thing to say. I have put on weight, but weight gain is a symptom of PCOS. I am the same woman and I still have feelings.'

When someone you don't know too well makes a comment such as, 'I thought you'd have had children by now. Don't you want them?' you could answer with, 'I would love to have children, but we don't always get what we want in life.' At this point the person will either be sympathetic, and you would have the chance of revealing more about your problems, if you wish, or the person may probe further, but in a way you find distasteful, saying, for instance, 'Aren't you doing it properly then?' It might be tempting to turn and flounce away at this juncture, but unfortunately you would probably be left with the feeling that the other person had got the upper hand and that you had allowed him or her to hurt you. Replying something to the effect of, 'Believe me, there's nothing I don't know about making babies – but actually I don't want to discuss this right now' will make you feel a little better.

Overcoming stress

Low self-esteem, persistent tiredness and anxiety about the future can cause a build-up of emotional stress. There are ways to help you develop a more positive outlook, however.

Living in the present

Women with PCOS would be well advised to try to live in the present. A calm and contented *now* is more emotionally nourishing than a mind reeling with the upsets the *future* may hold. In the same way, cherishing the moment is preferable to letting it slip by unappreciated because you are too busy thinking ahead. How many of us look forward to seeing a film, a band, a show, a play – but don't think to enjoy the journey there? How many of us look forward to summer, forgetting to appreciate spring? It is the same with numerous things in our lives.

But, you may ask, is it possible for someone who dislikes her appearance, who maybe is desperate to have children, to master the art of living in the present? But what is the alternative – to sit brooding on how things used to be, how they might now be, if only . . .? Wouldn't it be better to read a gripping book, pen a poem, surf the Internet, take a walk, or have a cuddle with that special someone? Admittedly, it is not always easy to lift bleak thoughts, but when you get into the habit of distracting yourself by turning to a pleasurable activity, it should eventually become second nature.

Accepting what you cannot change

There are many things in life that cannot be changed. Individuals can do nothing about the fact that they are either creative or practical, short-sighted or long-sighted, tall or short. Neither can you change the fact that you have PCOS – although you can certainly do many things to improve the situation. Acknowledging what you cannot change – and trying to live with it – is fundamental to stress management, for in accepting things as they are, you say goodbye to a great deal of frustration.

Finding new challenges

As well as offering distraction, taking on a new challenge can be infinitely rewarding and can help you to feel more positive about yourself. Consider taking up oil-painting, stencilling, playing the keyboard, tapestry-work, glass and china painting, picture-framing, jewellery-making ... the list is endless. The selection of 'things to do' in a craft shop alone is quite dazzling!

Learning something different can prove very satisfying. Maybe you might like to acquire a few academic qualifications, or take up a leisure interest course (where the atmosphere is more casual and regular attendance is not so important). Studying a subject that is helpful in dealing with PCOS (such as homoeopathy, reflexology, aromatherapy, meditation, relaxation, stress management or assertiveness training) may prove invaluable, too.

However, it is important that you choose an interest or study course that you will find stimulating and that you expect you'll do well at. Failure can be difficult to handle when you are also attempting to come to terms with the effects of the condition, or undergoing IVF treatments. Don't forget to congratulate yourself on each small success along the way.

Chronic stress

Chronic stress is the state of being constantly 'on alert'. The physiological changes associated with this state – a fast heart rate, shallow breathing and muscle tension – persist over a long period, making relaxation very difficult. Chronic stress can lead to nerviness, hypertension, irritability and depression.

The condition commonly arises when any of the following needs fail to be met on a long-term basis.

The need to be understood

Women with PCOS need to feel that the people close to them understand their concerns over their appearance and their worries over the long-term health risks that come with the condition. It is also of vital importance to them that family and close friends acknowledge their fears over whether or not they will be able to have children and, for those who are having problems conceiving, the myriad emotions that come with that.

When these people clearly believe you are worrying unnecessarily, you can feel so upset and isolated you begin to shut others out. Unfortunately, it is not always easy for others to understand how you feel. Taking a deep breath and calmly sharing your feelings is the most important step towards being understood and supported. However, if you have repeatedly tried to help them to understand and still they're upsetting you, tell them calmly how they are making you feel. Hopefully, this will shock them into seeing the situation from your point of view. If not, it would probably be more beneficial to your state of mind to cut yourself off from these people, if possible.

The need to be loved

Feeling unlovable is one of the greatest threats to the emotional well-being of women with PCOS. You may try to tell yourself that appearance isn't everything, yet concern that your partner now finds you unattractive – and so will ultimately end the relationship – may make you subconsciously withdraw your affections. You may even wonder how anyone *could* love you the way you look. The fear of being unlovable may even have caused you to become irrational and antagonistic.

Before you can be loved by others, you need to love yourself. You need to see yourself as a worthwhile person with qualities that you, as well as others, can respect. Don't let apathy rule. Start the way you mean to go on by taking the following action (some of these pointers have been mentioned earlier):

- make a list of your ten best physical attributes,
- make a list of your ten best character traits,
- do at least one nice thing (however small) for another person each day, and don't forget to congratulate yourself for it,
- make the very most of your appearance, every minute of the day,
- regularly treat yourself to a therapy that you find uplifting (for example, an aromatherapy or reflexology massage),
- try to indulge frequently in something that stimulates your mind while also creating a sense of fulfilment.

The need to love

PCOS can cause you to focus wholly on your symptoms, ultimately causing you to withdraw from the people around you. But loving others and actively attempting to lighten their mood can have a positive impact on your own state of mind. For example, encouraging your partner to smile will make you smile too; phoning a friend with relationship problems can make you feel useful and good about yourself, and showing interest in your lonely neighbour's vegetable patch can hearten you both. It doesn't need to take much, either. You can make someone smile with a few carefully chosen words – and a bit of honest flattery will make you feel just as good as the recipient. They are likely to be pleased and uplifted by the effort you have made, and, one hopes, will want to respond in kind. You have to give before you can hope to receive.

The need to be yourself

The roles many of us play out, perhaps unawares, often have their origins in early childhood. If, for example, the parents of a young woman – we'll call her Lisa – were always scathing of incompetence, she is likely to have grown up with the same mental attitude, going so far as to hide instances when she was less than perfect. Only when Lisa moves in with a partner who is far from perfect, a partner who may even be intimidated by her apparent 'perfection', will she begin to see that it is all right to be flawed.

There may be several ways in which you hide your real self. You may, for example, have dated a person who lived and breathed football. You liked this person a lot, so you read some of the sports pages and feigned an interest that you didn't actually feel. But, realistically, going through life pretending to be interested in something that you don't care a jot about causes untold inner stress. It is far better to be yourself, warts and all. This not only minimizes stress, it also ensures that you know that the people important to you like you for who you really are.

The need to feel well

Constantly being anxious and miserable can make a woman with PCOS feel unwell. Fatigue, intermittent pelvic pains and mood swings (for example – these may not be your particular symptoms) will only add to that feeling. However, taking positive steps to tackle the illness should help to counter the feeling of unwellness. For instance, you can improve matters by starting to eat healthily; taking regular exercise; avoiding exposure to harmful toxins; forging satisfactory relationships with your doctor, family and friends;

learning the art of positive thinking, and trying different complementary therapies. Whether or not the benefits are temporary, the feeling that you are actively helping yourself creates a sense of achievement and lowers stress levels.

Stress management

Because it is known that a woman with polycystic ovaries but no symptoms can develop the syndrome when subjected to a certain amount of stress, it is clear that stress is one of the triggering agents of PCOS.

Stress arises not only as a result of what happens to us, but also from our reactions to what happens. Negative inbred attitudes can actually cause people to see catastrophe in what to others would be normal, everyday events. When a situation is interpreted as a crisis, adrenaline is released into the bloodstream, and the body automatically puts itself 'on alert'. Breathing becomes shallow and fast, the heart rate quickens, blood pressure rises and the muscles tense – allowing the individual to deal with an emergency more effectively. This response can be destructive, however, when it occurs frequently, over a prolonged period of time.

Delay your reaction

Because living with a chronic condition naturally creates stress in daily life, women with PCOS experience higher levels of stress than non-sufferers. However, you should find that curbing your responses to certain occurrences can greatly reduce the build-up of stress. As a troublesome event unfolds, try not to react instantly. Allow yourself the time to evaluate the situation – to see it as it really is. Now select a response that doesn't create more stress.

Life stress evaluation

If you take the time to evaluate all the relationships and activities in your everyday life, you are likely to find some that induce a good deal more stress than benefit. Remember, however, that personal interactions will always produce a certain amount of stress. It is when the stress outweighs the positive gains that you need to consider limiting or ceasing that involvement.

Your relationships

Women with PCOS desperately need to know that the people close to them care. Most of all they crave the understanding of their nearest and dearest, feeling upset when they are shown thoughtlessness or impatience.

Partnerships

It is unfortunate that the distinctive problems experienced by women with PCOS are those that are most likely to intrude upon that most important relationship of all – their relationship with their partner. For a start, the premise that close partnerships should have no secrets is in peril, for who wants to tell her partner that she bleaches her facial hair and perhaps shaves around her nipples and navel? Unfortunately, regularly shutting yourself behind a locked door to do so can leave you feeling guilty. It may be equally difficult to admit to taking medication for acne.

Women deal with their PCOS in different ways. Most feel much better for opening up to their partners. Things that they had expected would shock their 'other half' generally only create a sense of empathy and strengthen that feeling of togetherness. It is possible that your partner had previously thought you were being secretive or that you were having mood swings because you were unhappy, but once a partner has been told the reason for these things, he usually tries to understand. Of course, your partner first has to discover how he himself actually feels.

If your partner really cares about you, he is likely to be concerned about the way you see yourself, your long-term health and how you might cope if you have difficulty conceiving. A small percentage of partners may, after some thought, decide these things are too much for them to handle and prefer to break up the relationship. It must be said, though, that this type of person would probably, in the long term, prove unsupportive and would possibly make you feel worse about yourself. Indeed, the relationship would probably have ended anyway at some point in the future.

Initiating a discussion on the subject can take a lot of courage, but it really is worth it. Try not to wait for that 'perfect moment' to start talking, either. Perfect moments never seem to arrive.

If your partner can't seem to understand your problems, the relationship may become a battleground, with each partner feeling resentful and unloved. Unless each makes an effort to understand the other person, the relationship may flounder. It is a fact that you can only truly know what your partner is thinking and feeling when you make time to talk problems through calmly. It is certainly worth the effort – for exchanging perceptions, fears and needs carries the bonus of strengthening your relationship.

However, if you have tried many times to discuss your problems calmly and still your partner refuses to understand, it does not bode well for the long-term success of the relationship. It's a fact that difficult relationships in themselves can be the reason for high stress levels and a failure to respond to treatment in women with PCOS.

Sex matters

Whether you are single or with a partner, sex is important. Women who are seeking a relationship need to be open to the prospect of sexual intimacy, and that is not always easy for someone with PCOS. Early on in a relationship, it is only human to try to hide areas that are less than perfect, and that includes excess facial or body hair, acne and perhaps certain areas of the body that you may think are too large or bumpy. Before each date you may scrupulously remove every offending hair, apply a thick coating of foundation and put on one of the two or three outfits that seems to miraculously give you a waist. It's not easy to keep this up, though, week after week, and sooner or later that special person will see a little more of how you really are. Once again, I suggest that as soon as the relationship starts to become serious, you try to open up about your problems.

Whether the relationship is still fairly new or you have been together for several years, women with PCOS can lose interest in sex. However, it's rarely the act itself they go off, rather they grow to dislike their body so much they can't bear to reveal it. It is only natural to want your partner to think you're attractive, but when you yourself feel you're anything but attractive, you may recoil at the idea of being seen naked or semi-naked.

The trouble is, if one partner – in this case the woman – appears to not want sex, the other may conclude that she's falling out of love and may start to doubt the strength of her feelings. If she then admits to not wanting sex because of her appearance, the partner will probably feel some relief and tell her she is worrying unnecessarily and that he still thinks her attractive. It is a fact that true love runs far deeper than physical appearance, even if your appearance was part of what attracted your partner in the first place. A person is rarely attracted solely by appearance. It also takes personality, shared interests and like-mindedness to make two people embark on a long-term relationship – at least, on one that stands a fair chance of succeeding.

If you are secure in the core strength of your relationship yet your sex life has dwindled, talking is undoubtedly the best way forward. Tell your partner you feel embarrassed to be seen naked or semi-naked, admit to not feeling very feminine, but end by telling your partner that you still love him. The most likely response will be reassurance that your partner still loves you and still wants to make love with you and that you have no need to feel embarrassed. A night of passion will then be on the cards, which you can prepare for as you wish. Try to make it extra special by lighting candles, by leading your partner to a soapy bath, by wearing that new sexy nightie . . .

If you really can't bring yourself to talk through your problems about sex with your partner, seeing a skilled relationship counsellor is perhaps your best course of action. That third sympathetic person may make it easier for you to admit to having problems with your appearance. If you think your problems are too embarrassing to speak so openly about, try joining an email chat room which deals with the subject. Alternatively, you could see a counsellor alone. This wouldn't be ideal, but a counsellor will try to give you the support and encouragement you need so you are able to speak to your partner.

Learning how to relax

Whether you are struggling to cope with the myriad symptoms of PCOS or undergoing IVF treatment, teaching yourself to relax can make all the difference to your stress levels.

Deep breathing
In normal breathing, we take oxygen from the atmosphere down into our lungs. The diaphragm contracts, and air is pulled into the chest cavity. When we breath out, we expel carbon dioxide and other

waste gases back into the atmosphere. But when we are stressed or upset, we tend to use the rib muscles to expand the chest. We breathe more quickly, sucking in shallowly. This is good in a crisis as it allows us to obtain the optimum amount of oxygen in the shortest possible time, providing our bodies with the extra power needed to handle the emergency.

Some people do tend to get stuck in chest-breathing mode. Long-term shallow breathing is not only detrimental to our physical and emotional health, it can also lead to hyperventilation, panic attacks, chest pains, dizziness and gastrointestinal problems.

To test your breathing, ask yourself:

- how fast are you breathing as you are reading this?
- are you pausing between breaths?
- are you breathing with your chest or with your diaphragm?

A breathing exercise

The following deep breathing exercise should, ideally, be performed daily.

- Lie down and make yourself comfortable in a warm room where you know you will be alone for at least half an hour.
- Close your eyes and try to relax.
- Gradually slow down your breathing, inhaling and exhaling as evenly as possible.
- Place one hand on your chest and the other on your abdomen, just below your rib cage.
- As you inhale, allow your abdomen to swell upwards. (Your chest should barely move.)
- As you exhale, let your abdomen fall and flatten.

Give yourself a few minutes to get into a smooth, easy rhythm. As worries and distractions arise, don't hang on to them. Wait calmly for them to float out of your mind – then focus once more on your breathing.

When you feel ready to end the exercise, open your eyes. Allow yourself time to become alert before rolling on to one side and getting up. With practice, you will begin breathing with your diaphragm quite naturally – and in times of stress, you should be able to correct your breathing without too much effort.

A relaxation exercise

Relaxation is one of the forgotten skills in today's hectic world. We already know that stress, which can give rise to insomnia, hypertension and depression, is one of the greatest enemies of the woman with PCOS. It is advisable, therefore, to learn at least one relaxation technique.

The following exercise is perhaps the easiest.

- Make yourself comfortable in a place where you will not be disturbed. Listening to restful music may help you to relax.
- Begin to slow down your breathing, inhaling through your nose to a count of two.
- Ensuring that the abdomen pushes outwards (as explained above), exhale to a count of four, five or six.
- After a couple of minutes, concentrate on each part of the body in turn, starting with your right arm. Consciously relax each set of muscles, allowing the tension to flow right out . . . Let your arm feel heavier and heavier as every last remnant of tension seeps away . . . Follow this procedure with the muscles of your left arm, then the muscles of your face, your neck, your stomach, your hips, and finally your legs.

Visualization

At this point, visualization can be introduced into the exercise. As you continue to breathe slowly and evenly, imagine yourself surrounded, perhaps, by lush, peaceful countryside, beside a gently trickling stream – or maybe on a deserted tropical beach, beneath swaying palm fronds, listening to the sounds of the ocean, thousands of miles from your worries and cares. Let the warm sun, the gentle breeze, the peacefulness of it all wash over you.

The tranquillity you feel at this stage can be enhanced by frequently repeating the exercise – once or twice a day is best. With time, you should be able to switch into a calm state of mind whenever you feel stressed.

Meditation

Arguably the oldest natural therapy, meditation is the simplest and most effective form of self-help. Ideally, the technique should be taught by a teacher – but, since meditation is essentially performed alone, it can be learned alone with equal success.

The unusual thing about meditation is that it involves 'letting go', allowing the mind to roam freely. However, as most of us are used to striving to control our thoughts, letting go is not so easy as it sounds.

It may help you to know that people who regularly meditate say they have more energy, require less sleep, are less anxious, and feel far more 'alive' than before they did so. Studies have shown that during meditation the heart rate slows, blood pressure reduces, and the circulation improves, making the hands and feet feel much warmer.

Meditation may, to some people, sound a bit off-beat. But isn't it worth a try – especially when you can do it for free! Kick off those shoes and make yourself comfortable, somewhere you can be alone for a while. Now follow these simple instructions.

- Close your eyes, relax, and practise the deep breathing exercise as described above.
- Concentrate on your breathing. Try to free your mind of conscious control. Letting it roam unchecked, try to allow the deeper, more serene part of you to take over.
- If you wish to go further into meditation, concentrate now on mentally repeating a mantra – a certain word or phrase. It should be something positive, such as 'relax', 'I feel calm' or 'I am a very special person'.
- When you are ready to finish, open your eyes and allow time to adjust to the outside world before getting to your feet.

The aim of mentally repeating a mantra is to plant the positive thought into your subconscious mind. It is a form of self-hypnosis, only you alone control the messages placed there.

Useful Addresses

PCOS support group

Verity
52–54 Featherstone Street
London EC1Y 8RT
Tel. 020 7251 9009
Email <enquiries@verity-pcos.org.uk>
Website <http://www.verity-pcos.org.uk>
Verity is a national PCOS support group

Complementary treatment

British Acupuncture Council
63 Jeddo Road
London W12 9HQ
Tel 020 8735 0400
Email <info@acupuncture.org.uk>
Website <http://www.acupuncture.org.uk>

Depression

Depression Alliance
35 Westminster Bridge Road
London SE1 7JB
Tel. 020 7633 0557
Email <information@depressionalliance.org>
Website <http://www.depressionalliance.org>

Diabetes

Diabetes UK (formerly the British Diabetic Association)
10 Parkway
London NW1 7AA
Tel. 020 7424 1000
Email<info@diabetes.org.uk>
Website <http://www.diabetes.org.uk>

Eating Disorders

Eating Disorder Recovery
Email <jrust@edrecovery.com>
Website <http://www.edrecovery.com>

Eating Disorders Association
103 Prince of Wales Road
Norwich
Norfolk NR1 1DW
Tel. 0845 634 1414
Email <info@edauk.com>
Website <http://www.edauk.com>

Tottenham Women's Health Centre
15 Fenhurst Gate
Aughton, Ormskirk
Lancs L39 5ED

Fertility and adoption

BAAF Adoption and Fostering
Skyline House
200 Union Street
London SE1 0LX
Tel. 020 7593 2000
Email <mail@baaf.org.uk>
Website <http://www.baaf.org.uk>

British Fertility Society Secretariat
22 Apex Court
Woodlands
Bradley Stoke BS32 4NQ
Tel. 01454 642217
Email <bfs@bioscientifica.com>
Website <http://www.britishfertilitysociety.org.uk>
The British Fertility Society is a national society for healthcare professionals

British Infertility Counselling Association (BICA)
69 Division Street
Sheffield S1 4GE
Tel. 0114 263 1448
Website <http://www.bica.net>

CHILD
Charter House
43 St Leonards Road,
Bexhill-on-Sea
East Sussex TN40 1JA
Tel. 01424 732361
Email <office@child.org.uk>
Website <http://www.child.org.uk>
CHILD is a national support organization with newsletter and helpline

Human Fertilisation and Embryology Authority (HFEA)
Paxton House
30 Artillery Lane
London E1 7LS
Tel. 020 7377 5077
Email <http://admin@hfea.gov.uk>
Website <http://www.hfea.gov.uk>

Issue
114 Lichfield Street
Walsall WS1 1SZ
Tel. 01922 722888
Email <info@issue.co.uk>
Website <http://www.issue.co.uk>
Issue is a national fertility support organization

Miscarriage Association
c/o Clayton Hospital
Northgate
Wakefield WF1 3JS
Tel. 01924 200799
Email <info@miscarriageassociation.org.uk>
Website <http://www.miscarriageassociation.org.uk>

Multiple Births Foundation
Hammersmith House Level 4
Queen Charlotte's & Chelsea Hospital
Du Cane Road
London W12 0HS
Tel. 020 8383 3519
Email <info@multiplebirths.org.uk>
Website <http://www.multiplebirths.org.uk

Food and nutrition

BioCare Ltd
Lakeside
180 Lifford Lane
Kings Norton
Birmingham B30 3NU
Tel. 0121 433 3727 (sales, orders and enquiries)
Tel. 0121 433 8702 (technical enquiries)
Fax 0121 433 8705 (sales and orders)
Email <biocare@biocare.co.uk>
Website <http://www.biocare.co.uk>
For high quality practitioner-grade supplements

British Nutrition Foundation
High Holborn House
52–54 High Holborn
London WC1V 6RQ
Tel. 020 7404 6504
Email <postbox@nutrition.org.uk>
Website <http://www.nutrition.org.uk>

The Nutri Centre
7 Park Crescent
London W1B 1PF
Tel. 020 7436 5122 (supplement orders and professional advice)
Fax 020 7436 5171
Email <enq@nutricentre.com>
Website <http://www.nutricentre.com>
For good quality supplements, and subscription to the regular
NutriNews publication

The Nutrition Mission
6 Havelocks
Crook Farm
Glen Road
Baildon
Shipley BD17 6ED
Tel. 01725 514222 (ordering)
Tel. 01274 590383 (consultations)
Email <info@nutrition-mission.co.uk>
Website <http://www.nutrition-mission.co.uk>
For an excellent one-a-day high antioxidant containing over 30 ingredients including the B vitamins, high-dose pantothenic acid and omega-3 and omega-6 essential fatty acids, liver support (which gets the liver and gall bladder working properly so that toxins are expelled) and intestinal tone (which balances the gut flora and removes toxins from the body, helping to ease constipation or diarrhoea, flatulence and bloating)

Simply Organic Food Company Ltd
Horsley Road
Kingsthorpe Hollow
Northampton NN2 6LJ
Tel. 0870 760 6001 (to place an order)
Tel. 01604 791911 (other customer enquiries)
Fax 01604 718049
Email <orders@simplyorganic.net>
Website: <http://www.simplyorganic.net>
For fresh, organic produce. Online or telephone ordering. Brochure available on request.

The Soil Association
Bristol House
40–56 Victoria Street
Bristol BS1 6BY
Tel. 0117 929 0661
Email <info@soilassociation.org.uk>
Website <http://www.soilassociation.org.uk>

Skin and hair

Acne Support Group
PO Box 9
Newquay
Cornwall TR9 6WG
Tel. 0870 870 2263
Website <http://www.m2w3.com/acne>

Follicle.com
Website <http://www.follicle.com/types>

Hairline International – The Alopecia Patients Society
Lyons Court
1668 High Street
Knowle
West Midlands B93 0LY
Tel. 01564 775281
Website <http://www.hairlineinternational.com>

References

1 I. F. Stein and M. L. Leventhal, 'Amenorrhea associated with bilateral polycystic ovaries', *American Journal of Obstetrics and Gynecology*, 1935, 29, pp. 181–91.

2 A. H. Balen, 'The pathogenesis of polycystic ovary syndrome: the enigma unravels', *Lancet*, 1999, 354, pp. 966–7.

3 A. H. Balen, G. S. Conway, G. Kaltsas, K. Techatraisak, P. J. Manning, C. West and H. S. Lisas, 'PCOS: the spectrum of the disorder in 1741 patients', *Human Reproduction*, 1995, 10, pp. 2705–12.

4 S. Franks, N. Gharani, D. Waterworth, S. Batty, D. White, R. Williamson and M. McCarthy, 'The genetic basis of polycystic ovary syndrome', *Human Reproduction*, 1997, 12, pp. 2641–8.

5 Franks and others, 'The genetic basis of polycystic ovary syndrome'.

6 D. M. Waterworth, S. T. Bennett, N. Gharani, M. McCarthy, S. Hague, S. Batty, G. S. Conway, D. White, J. A. Todd, S. Franks and R. Williamson, 'Linkage and association of insulin gene VNTR regulatory polymorphism with PCOS', *Lancet*, 1997, 349, pp. 1771–2.

7 A. Dunaif, 'Insulin resistance and the polycystic ovary syndrome: mechanisms and implication for pathogenesis', *Endocrine Review*, 1997, 18, pp. 774–800.

8 G. S. Conway, 'Insulin resistance and PCOS', *Contemporary Review in Obstetrics and Gynaecology*, 1990, 2, pp. 34–9.

9 P. Acien, F. Quereda, P. Matallin, E. Villarroya, J. A. Lopez-Fernandez, M. Acien, M. Mauri and R. Alfayate, 'Insulin, androgens and obesity in women with and without PCOS, a heterogenous group of disorders', *Fertility and Sterility*, 1999, 72, pp. 32–40.

10 J. E. Nestler and D. J. Jakubowics, 'Decreases in ovarian cytochrome P450c 17 alpha activity and serum free testosterone after reduction of insulin secretion in polycystic ovary syndrome', *New England Journal of Medicine*, 1996, 335, pp. 617–23.

11 E. M. Velazquez, A. Acosta and S. G. Mendoza, 'Menstrual

cyclicity after metformin therapy in PCOS', *Obstetrics and Gynecology*, 1997, 90, pp. 392–5.

12 L. C. Morin-Papunen, R. M. Koivunen, A. Ruokonen and H. K. Martikainen, 'Metformin therapy improves the menstrual pattern with minimal endocrine and metabolic effects in women with PCOS', *Fertility and Sterility*, 1998, 69, pp. 691–6.

13 J. E. Nestler, D. J. Jakubowics, W. S. Evans and R. Pasquali, 'Effects of metformin on spontaneous ovulation an clomiphene-induced ovulation in PCOS', *New England Journal of Medicine*, 1998, 338, pp. 1876–80.

14 A. H. Balen, D. D. M. Braat, C. West, A. Patel and H. S. Lisas, 'Cumulative conception and live birth rates after the treatment of anovulatory infertility. An analysis of the safety and efficacy of ovulation induction in 200 patients', *Human Reproduction*, 1994, 9, pp. 1563–70.

15 A. Abden Gadir, R. S. Mowafi, H. M. I. Alnaser, A. H. Alrashid, O. M. Alonezi and R. W. Shaw, 'Ovarian electrocautery versus human menopausal gonadotrophins and pure follicle stimulating hormone therapy in the treatment of patients with PCOS', *Clinical Endocrinology*, 1990, 33, pp. 585–92.

16 R. H. Hall, 'The agri-business view of soil and life', *Journal of Holistic Medicine*, 1981, 3, pp. 157–66.

17 F. Goldstein, M. B. Goldman, L. Ryan and D. W. Cramer, 'Relation of female infertility to consumption of caffeinated beverages', *American Journal of Epidemiology*, 1993, 137, pp. 1353–60.

18 K. Kupparanjan, 'Effect of Ashwagandha on the process of ageing in human volunteers', *Journal of Research in Ayurveda and Sadai*, 1980, pp. 247–58.

Further Reading

Angie Best-Boss, *Living with PCOS*, Addicus, Omaha, Nebraska, USA, 2001.

Dr Joan Gomez, *Living with Diabetes*, Sheldon Press, London, 1998.

Colette Harris and Dr Adam Carey, *PCOS: A Woman's Guide to Dealing with Polycystic Ovary Syndrome*, HarperCollins, London, 2000.

Colette Harris and Theresa Francis Cheung, *PCOS Diet Book: How You Can Use the Nutritional Approach to Deal with Polycystic Ovary Syndrome*, HarperCollins, London, 2002.

Patrick Holford, *The Optimum Nutrition Bible*, Piatkus, London, 1998.

Patrick Holford and Kate Neil, *Balancing Hormones Naturally*, Piatkus, London, 1998.

Elizabeth Holmes, *The Natural Way: Acne*, HarperCollins, London, 2000.

Leslie Kenton, *The Raw Energy Bible*, Vermilion, London, 2001.

Cheryl Kimball and Milton Hammerly, *What to do when the doctor says it's PCOS: Polycystic Ovary Syndrome: The Most Important Things You Need to Know*, Fair Winds Press, Rockport, Massachusetts, USA, 2003.

Index